CertiPrep – CMA (AAMA) Exam Prep Book 2025–2026

CertiPrep

Published by CertiPrep Publishing, 2025.

CERTIPREP – CMA (AAMA) EXAM PREP BOOK 2025–2026

First edition. November 11, 2025.

ISBN: 979-8232438227

Written by CertiPrep.

Table of Contents

Disclaimer

This book is an independent study resource created to help candidates prepare for the CMA (AAMA)® Certification Exam. It is **not** sponsored, endorsed, or approved by the American Association of Medical Assistants (AAMA)® or any other organization.

The Certifying Board of the AAMA may update eligibility criteria, exam policies, the Content Outline, and scoring procedures at any time. You are responsible for reviewing the most current information on the official AAMA website—especially the CMA (AAMA)® Certification Exam application, content outline, and preparation materials—before you sit for the exam.

Every reasonable effort has been made to ensure accuracy at the time of writing, but the authors and publisher cannot guarantee that all information will remain current or error-free. Using this book does **not** guarantee a passing score. Your results will depend on your education, clinical and administrative experience, and how you study.

"Certified Medical Assistant (AAMA)®," "CMA (AAMA)®," "American Association of Medical Assistants®," and related marks are registered trademarks of the American Association of Medical Assistants. This book is independent of the AAMA and is not sponsored, endorsed, or affiliated with the Association.

About This Book

THIS CERTIPREP GUIDE is designed to feel like your other exam prep books: conversational, practical, and tightly aligned to the actual exam content. Instead of drowning you in lists, it focuses on realistic CMA tasks and turns them into exam-style questions and explanations.

Chapters are broken into small, focused sections you can study in 15–20 minutes. Each section gives you a quick overview, a few high-yield bullet points, and a deeper dive so you can understand not just **what** to do, but **why** the exam matters. Every chapter ends with practice questions and rationales to reinforce the most testable ideas.

CMA (AAMA) Exam Snapshot

THE CMA (AAMA) EXAM is a computer-based test with **200 multiple-choice questions**, including scored and unscored items. You'll have a total of **3 hours** to complete these questions across the exam's timed segments.

Questions are built from a detailed content outline published by the AAMA. The outline groups tested knowledge and skills into three main domains: **Clinical**, **General**, and **Administrative**. Clinical content is the largest portion of the exam, but General and Administrative topics still make up a substantial share, so a balanced study plan is essential.

Who This Book Is For

THIS BOOK IS WRITTEN for candidates who are currently in—or have recently completed—a medical assisting program, as well as working MAs who are ready to earn the CMA (AAMA) credential. It assumes you have basic familiarity with medical terminology, anatomy and physiology, and routine clinical and office procedures.

You do **not** need years of experience to use this guide. Explanations begin at a practical level, then build toward exam-style reasoning. If you have hands-on experience, the scenarios will feel familiar; if you're newer, they'll give you a realistic preview of your role.

How to Use This Book

YOU CAN USE THIS BOOK as a complete study course or as a structured review in the final weeks before your exam. Start by reading each chapter section, then immediately work through the related practice questions and review the rationales.

After you complete the content chapters, take the full-length practice exam in one sitting under timed conditions. Your performance will highlight which domains you've mastered and which still need work, allowing you to target your limited study time where it matters most.

Book Overview

Chapter 1

CMA Exam Overview and Medical Assisting Fundamentals

This chapter lays the foundation for the entire CMA (AAMA) exam. You'll learn what the credential represents, how the exam is structured, and what kind of thinking the exam expects from a professional medical assistant. The goal is to help you see the "big picture" so that later clinical and administrative details make sense instead of feeling random.

1.1 The CMA (AAMA) Credential and Exam Basics

THE CMA (AAMA) IS A nationally recognized credential that validates your competency as a multi-skilled medical assistant. The exam that leads to this credential is carefully structured and standardized to give all candidates a fair assessment of their knowledge and skills.

- Nationally recognized credential proving multi-skilled competence
- Computer-based multiple-choice exam with a fixed time limit
- Content organized into clearly defined domains

The CMA (AAMA) credential signals to employers that you've completed formal training and passed a rigorous exam, not just picked up skills informally on the job. It shows you have a solid foundation in patient care, communication, and office operations. Because it's nationally recognized, it can improve your employment opportunities across different states and practice settings. Many employers either prefer or require CMA (AAMA) certification for hiring or advancement.

The exam itself is administered on a computer at approved testing centers or remotely in controlled environments. All questions are multiple-choice, which allows standardized scoring and consistent difficulty from candidate to candidate. You'll have a strictly limited amount of time, so pacing is part of your test-taking skill set. Understanding this structure helps you practice under realistic conditions instead of casually flipping through questions.

The CMA (AAMA) content is divided into explicit domains so the exam can measure specific areas consistently. This content outline is public, and you should treat it as your "map" while studying. When an exam uses defined domains, it's less about tricking you and more about confirming you meet clear standards. If you use the domains to plan your studying, you'll be working with the exam instead of guessing what might show up.

1.2 Where CMAs Work and Core Responsibilities

CERTIFIED MEDICAL ASSISTANTS work in many outpatient environments, but the essential tasks they perform remain consistent. Knowing where CMAs are commonly employed helps you relate exam scenarios to realistic settings. Understanding your core responsibilities keeps you focused on what matters most on test day and on the job.

- Typical outpatient and clinic settings for CMAs
- Core responsibilities that follow you from job to job

Most CMA (AAMA) certificants work in physician offices, multi-specialty clinics, and outpatient departments rather than inpatient hospital units. The exam frequently uses examples from family practice, pediatrics, internal medicine, and specialty offices like cardiology or obstetrics to make questions feel familiar. Even if you currently work in one specific area, the test expects you to function safely in any typical ambulatory setting. Keeping these environments in mind while studying helps you imagine what the "room" looks like in each scenario.

Core responsibilities include preparing patients for exams, collecting and documenting accurate data, assisting with procedures, and keeping both the clinical and administrative workflow running smoothly. You might move from taking vital signs to managing a phone call or scheduling a follow-up in a single encounter. The exam reflects this by mixing clinical and office tasks within one question. When you see a scenario, always ask yourself how a competent CMA would manage both the patient and the paperwork at the same time.

1.3 The Three Exam Domains: Clinical, General, Administrative

THE CMA (AAMA) EXAM is built around three primary domains that mirror your role in real practice. Clinical content receives the largest emphasis, but General and Administrative domains are essential for safe and effective care. Understanding how these domains interact guides your study plan and your approach to questions.

- Clinical domain: hands-on patient care and procedures
- General domain: foundational knowledge and professional behavior
- Administrative domain: front-office operations and basic financial processes

The Clinical domain covers tasks like infection control, vital signs, specimen collection, diagnostic tests, and assisting with procedures. These are the skills you use when you are physically in the exam room or treatment area with a patient. In exam questions, clinical content often shows up as a sequence of steps or as a decision about what action to take next. To answer correctly, you must know both what to do and in what order to do it.

The General domain includes anatomy and physiology, pathophysiology, psychology, and communication, as well as legal and ethical considerations. This domain forms the background knowledge that makes your clinical actions make sense. For example, understanding how the cardiovascular system works helps you recognize when vital signs are abnormal. Ethical and legal questions in this domain check that you respect patient rights and professional boundaries while you carry out tasks.

The Administrative domain focuses on front-office duties such as reception, scheduling, records management, billing, and basic coding. While these tasks may not feel as "clinical," they are critical to keeping the practice functioning and ensuring patients receive timely, organized care. On the exam, administrative questions often test attention to detail, organization, and professionalism in communication. A strong CMA is not only safe in the exam room but also competent at the desk and in the EHR.

1.4 Scope of Practice and Delegation

SCOPE OF PRACTICE DEFINES what a CMA is allowed and trained to do, while delegation describes how providers and licensed nurses assign tasks to you. The exam frequently tests whether you understand where your authority ends and the provider's authority begins. Staying inside your scope protects patients, your employer, and your certification.

- CMA scope versus provider and nurse responsibilities

- Delegated tasks and the need for supervision

CMA (AAMA) certificants are trained to collect data, perform certain clinical procedures, and educate patients within defined limits. You are not authorized to diagnose conditions, prescribe medications, or independently decide to change a patient's treatment plan. On exam questions, answers that invite you to "act like the provider" are usually incorrect. Instead, the safest option is the one where you support the provider's plan and accurately report information.

Delegation means that a licensed provider or nurse assigns tasks to you that are within your training and legal scope. Even when tasks are delegated, the delegating provider retains overall responsibility for patient care. Your responsibility is to perform the delegated task exactly as instructed and report back anything significant. On the exam, when a task seems beyond your training, the correct response is usually to notify the provider or nurse rather than improvising.

1.5 Safety and Infection Control Fundamentals

SAFETY AND INFECTION control are at the heart of safe patient care and a major focus of the CMA exam. Many questions are essentially asking you to choose the safest, most responsible action. If you consistently think "safety first," you will often find the best answer.

- Standard Precautions for all patients
- Hand hygiene, PPE, and sharps safety

Standard Precautions are infection-control practices that apply to every patient, regardless of their known or suspected diagnosis. They assume that all blood and certain body fluids may carry infectious agents. This concept shows up on the exam when you decide whether gloves, masks, or other measures are needed. Even if a patient appears healthy, Standard Precautions still apply because infection status is not always obvious.

Hand hygiene is considered the single most important way to prevent the spread of infection. You should perform hand hygiene before and after patient contact, after removing gloves, and after contact with potentially contaminated surfaces. Personal protective equipment (PPE) such as gloves, masks, gowns, or eye protection should be used according to the task and the risk of exposure. Safe sharps handling includes never recapping needles, disposing of sharps immediately in approved containers, and reporting any needle-stick injury. On the exam, any answer that cuts corners on these basics—even in a "busy clinic" scenario—is almost always wrong.

1.6 Communication and Patient Interaction

GOOD COMMUNICATION is a core skill for CMAs and is tested heavily on the exam. The questions often use short scenarios to see how you would talk with patients, families, and the healthcare team. Your answers should reflect professionalism, clarity, and respect.

- Introducing yourself and explaining procedures in plain language
- Using therapeutic communication strategies

When you enter the room, you're expected to introduce yourself by name and role, verify the patient's identity, and briefly explain what you're about to do. This builds trust and helps reduce anxiety, especially for patients who are nervous or unsure why they are there. Using plain language instead of unexplained medical jargon makes your explanations more effective. The exam tends to reward answers that make the patient feel informed and included.

Therapeutic communication includes skills like active listening, reflection, and empathy. Instead of judging or criticizing, you invite the patient to share more about what they are experiencing. Phrases like "Tell me more about..." or "It sounds like you're feeling..." are often better than "Why didn't you...?" or "You should have...". On exam questions, the best response is usually the one that acknowledges the patient's feelings and keeps the conversation open, not the one that shuts it down or makes the patient feel blamed.

1.7 Legal, Ethical, and Confidentiality Basics

LEGAL AND ETHICAL PRINCIPLES give structure to your everyday actions as a CMA. You do not need to memorize every law, but you must understand the main ideas and how they show up in typical office situations. Confidentiality is a recurring theme and an easy way to lose points if you're careless.

- Protecting patient privacy and confidentiality
- Accurate documentation, consent, and release of information

Protecting privacy means handling patient information in a way that keeps it secure and only shared with authorized individuals. This includes not discussing patients in hallways, elevators, or waiting rooms where others can overhear. It also means being careful with computer screens, paper charts, and phone calls. Exam scenarios often present a choice between convenience and confidentiality; the correct answer always errs on the side of protecting the patient's information.

Accurate documentation is both a legal and ethical requirement. You should chart objective facts, avoid altering records to hide errors, and follow the facility's process for making corrections. Consent, particularly informed consent, involves explaining procedures, risks, and benefits so patients can make decisions about their care. Release of information requires proper authorization before sending records to third parties. On the exam, answers that involve falsifying information, sharing records without permission, or ignoring clear policy are almost always wrong.

1.8 Clinical vs. Administrative Thinking in Scenarios

MANY CMA QUESTIONS blend clinical and administrative work into a single situation. Your job is to untangle what needs to happen clinically and what needs to happen administratively, then prioritize appropriately. This is where your understanding of the three domains becomes practical.

- Recognizing clinical tasks versus administrative tasks in a scenario
- Prioritizing safety and confidentiality while managing workflow

Clinical tasks include things like measuring vital signs, preparing exam rooms, assisting with procedures, and documenting in the medical record. Administrative tasks cover greeting patients, scheduling, answering phones, handling basic billing questions, and managing forms. In real life, you switch between these roles constantly, and the exam mimics this reality. Identifying which parts of the scenario are clinical and which are administrative helps you choose the step that makes the most sense.

When both clinical and administrative issues compete for your attention, you must prioritize. Patient safety and confidentiality should always come first, even if it means asking someone else to help at the front desk or briefly delaying a phone call. For example, you would not leave a patient on the exam table unattended to answer a non-urgent scheduling question. Exam questions often reward the answer that protects the patient in the room and manages other tasks in a calm, professional way afterward.

1.9 How CMA Questions Are Built

CMA EXAM QUESTIONS may look straightforward, but they're carefully designed to test judgment, not just memorization. Instead of asking you to recite definitions, they put those definitions into situations that require you to choose the best action. Learning to recognize common patterns in question design will help you work more confidently.

- Scenario-based multiple-choice questions
- Key wording such as "FIRST," "BEST," and "MOST appropriate"

Most questions provide a short scenario followed by four answer choices. Often, more than one option seems somewhat reasonable, but only one is clearly the safest and most professional. The exam expects you to apply your knowledge to a situation rather than treating each fact in isolation. This is why simply memorizing lists without understanding can leave you stuck between two possible answers.

Words like "FIRST," "BEST," or "MOST appropriate" are crucial because they tell you what the test is truly asking. "First" usually refers to immediate safety or assessment before long-term solutions. "Best" and "most appropriate" hint that there may be several acceptable actions, but one stands out as the safest, most ethical, or most efficient. Wrong answers often break safety rules, ignore scope of practice, or reveal confidential information, even if they solve part of the problem. Training yourself to spot these traps will improve your accuracy.

1.10 Smart Study Strategies for This Exam

A STRONG STUDY PLAN can make the difference between barely passing and feeling confident on exam day. Instead of passively reading, you should actively test yourself and adjust your study focus as you go. The goal is to make the CMA exam feel familiar by the time you sit down to take it.

- Build a study plan around the three exam domains
- Use practice questions to find and fix weak areas

Start by reviewing the official content outline and mapping your study time to the percentage of questions in each domain. Since Clinical is the largest, it deserves more hours, but you still need solid coverage of General and Administrative topics. Breaking chapters into daily or weekly goals makes the workload more manageable. It also helps prevent last-minute cramming, which is less effective for long-term retention.

Practice questions are one of your most powerful tools. Each time you miss a question, you've found a specific concept that needs attention. After reviewing the explanation, go back to the related section in the text and reread it with that question in mind. Over time, you will see patterns in what you miss—maybe infection control steps or documentation rules—and you can spend extra time on those themes. This targeted approach is far more efficient than reading everything over and over.

Practice Questions – Chapter 1 (25 Questions)

THESE QUESTIONS FOCUS on the concepts from Chapter 1: the CMA credential, exam structure, domains, scope of practice, safety fundamentals, communication, legal/ethical basics, and study strategy.

1. The **main purpose** of the CMA (AAMA) credential is to:
   A. Grant medical assistants the legal authority to diagnose patients
   B. Verify that a medical assistant has met a national standard of knowledge and skill
   C. Replace all state regulations governing medical assistants
   D. Allow medical assistants to practice independently without supervision
2. Which statement best describes the **format** of the CMA (AAMA) exam?
   A. A written essay exam with oral interviews
   B. A computer-based exam made up of multiple-choice questions
   C. A hands-on skills test with no written component
   D. A take-home open-book exam
3. The primary reason the exam is divided into Clinical, General, and Administrative domains is to:
   A. Make the test longer and more difficult
   B. Allow candidates to choose which domain they want to be tested on
   C. Ensure that all key areas of a medical assistant's role are assessed
   D. Focus only on clinical tasks while ignoring office skills
4. Which setting is **most typical** for a CMA (AAMA) certificant?
   A. Intensive care unit in a hospital
   B. Outpatient physician office or clinic
   C. Long-term care nursing home
   D. Home health agency
5. Which task is **clearly within** the CMA scope of practice?
   A. Prescribing an antibiotic for a suspected infection
   B. Changing a patient's medication dose when symptoms worsen
   C. Collecting a blood pressure and documenting it in the EHR
   D. Diagnosing a patient with hypertension
6. A provider delegates a task to the CMA. Which statement is most accurate?
   A. The CMA becomes solely responsible for all outcomes of that task
   B. The provider retains overall responsibility, and the CMA must perform the task as instructed
   C. The CMA may alter the task based on personal preference
   D. Delegation allows the CMA to perform any procedure they choose
7. Standard Precautions are designed to:
   A. Be used only for patients with known infections
   B. Apply to all patients, regardless of infection status
   C. Replace the need for hand hygiene
   D. Eliminate the need for PPE
8. Which action best follows Standard Precautions?
   A. Recapping used needles to prevent accidental sticks
   B. Disposing of used sharps immediately in an approved sharps container
   C. Placing used needles in a regular trash can if the sharps container is full

D. Leaving used sharps on a tray until the end of the shift

9. A CMA prepares to enter an exam room. Which action shows **good communication** practice?
   A. Walking in without knocking and starting the procedure
   B. Introducing themselves by name and role and confirming the patient's identity
   C. Rushing the explanation because the schedule is behind
   D. Using complex medical terminology to sound professional
10. Which is the **best example** of therapeutic communication?
   A. "Why didn't you follow the instructions we gave you?"
   B. "You should have called us sooner."
   C. "It sounds like you've been really worried. Can you tell me more about what's been happening?"
   D. "If you don't change your habits, you're going to get worse."
11. A CMA is discussing a patient's test results in a hallway where others can hear. This behavior:
   A. Is acceptable if the discussion is brief
   B. Violates patient confidentiality
   C. Is allowed as long as no names are used
   D. Is encouraged to save time
12. Which action best protects **patient privacy** at the front desk?
   A. Asking patients to state their chief complaint loudly
   B. Calling patients by full name and diagnosis in the waiting room
   C. Speaking quietly and avoiding detailed discussions of medical issues in public areas
   D. Leaving patient charts open on the counter
13. A CMA notices an error in a blood pressure reading entered into the EHR. What should the CMA do?
   A. Ignore it because it is only one reading
   B. Delete the record so no one sees the mistake
   C. Correct the entry according to facility policy, documenting the correction clearly
   D. Change the reading silently without noting any correction
14. A patient asks the CMA, "Do I have pneumonia?" after an exam. What is the **best** response?
   A. "Yes, you definitely have pneumonia."
   B. "No, you definitely do not have pneumonia."
   C. "That's something the provider will diagnose. I'll let them know you have questions so they can explain your results."
   D. "Let's search online together and see what it says."
15. A question on the exam asks what the CMA should do **first** in a scenario. This usually means you should:
   A. Choose the action that is fastest
   B. Look for the step that maximizes clinic revenue
   C. Identify the safest initial step that protects the patient
   D. Pick the option that avoids contacting the provider
16. Which of the following behaviors in a busy clinic is **most appropriate**?
   A. Skipping hand hygiene between patients to stay on schedule
   B. Asking another staff member for help so infection-control standards are maintained
   C. Leaving sharps to dispose of later when things calm down
   D. Discussing patient cases in the waiting room to speed decisions
17. The Administrative domain of the exam focuses mainly on:
   A. Surgical technique and wound care

B. Reception, scheduling, records, billing, and basic coding
C. Pharmacology and drug interactions
D. Nutrition counseling and meal planning

18. Which study strategy is **most effective** for preparing for the CMA exam?
A. Reading the textbook cover to cover without answering questions
B. Using practice questions to identify weak areas and then reviewing those topics
C. Waiting until the week before the exam to start studying
D. Only studying topics you already feel comfortable with
19. During a practice test, a candidate misses several questions about scope of practice. What should they do?
A. Ignore those questions and hope they don't appear on the real exam
B. Focus only on clinical procedures and forget legal topics
C. Review scope-of-practice content and redo similar practice questions
D. Switch to a different exam entirely
20. On the job, which action most closely matches what the CMA exam will expect?
A. Acting independently to adjust medications based on personal judgment
B. Following facility policies, documenting accurately, and staying within scope
C. Avoiding communication with providers to stay out of trouble
D. Skipping PPE if the patient appears "healthy"
21. A CMA is rooming a patient when the front desk calls with a scheduling question. Which is the most appropriate action?
A. Leave the patient on the exam table to handle the scheduling issue immediately
B. Finish the essential clinical tasks with the patient safely, then respond to the scheduling issue
C. Ask the patient to answer the scheduling question to save time
D. Ignore the front desk and hope they call someone else
22. A practice question asks what is the "most appropriate" CMA response to a frustrated patient. You should:
A. Choose the answer that avoids extra work
B. Pick the response that uses therapeutic communication and respects the patient
C. Select the option that changes the subject quickly
D. Choose the response that tells the patient they are overreacting
23. Which action is the **best example** of aligning with the General domain of the exam?
A. Understanding how hypertension affects the cardiovascular system
B. Calculating insurance reimbursements
C. Cleaning instruments in an autoclave
D. Scheduling follow-up appointments
24. Why is it important to know that the Clinical domain has the largest weight on the exam?
A. So you can study only Clinical and ignore everything else
B. So you can decide not to learn Administrative tasks
C. So you can give Clinical extra study time while still covering General and Administrative topics
D. So you can guess on all Clinical questions and focus on the rest
25. During the real exam, a candidate finishes a block of questions with ten minutes left. What is the **best** use of that time?
A. Sit and wait without touching any answers
B. Randomly change answers to different choices
C. Review marked questions and check for misread words, safety issues, or scope violations

D. Close the exam section early because they feel confident

Answer Key – Chapter 1 (with Justifications)

1. **B** – The CMA (AAMA) credential exists to show that a medical assistant has met a national standard of knowledge and skills across clinical, administrative, and general areas, not to grant independent diagnostic authority.
2. **B** – The exam is delivered on the computer as a multiple-choice test, which allows standardized administration and scoring.
3. **C** – Dividing the exam into domains ensures that the test measures all major aspects of the MA role, including clinical, general knowledge, and administrative skills.
4. **B** – CMAs typically work in outpatient offices and clinics; this is the setting most frequently reflected in exam scenarios.
5. **C** – Collecting and documenting vital signs is a standard CMA task, while diagnosing or prescribing medications is outside scope and reserved for licensed providers.
6. **B** – When a provider delegates a task, they maintain overall responsibility, and the CMA must perform the task as directed within their training and scope.
7. **B** – Standard Precautions are designed to be used with all patients, because infection status is not always known.
8. **B** – Used sharps must be placed immediately into an approved sharps container; recapping or using regular trash is unsafe and violates sharps safety standards.
9. **B** – Introducing yourself by name and role and confirming the patient's identity reflects professional, patient-centered communication.
10. **C** – This response acknowledges the patient's feelings, invites them to share more, and uses therapeutic communication rather than blame or criticism.
11. **B** – Discussing patient information in a hallway where others can overhear violates confidentiality and is not acceptable practice.
12. **C** – Speaking quietly and avoiding detailed discussions of medical issues in public areas helps protect patient privacy at the front desk.
13. **C** – The proper action is to correct the error following policy and document the correction; hiding or ignoring the mistake is unethical and unsafe.
14. **C** – Diagnosing is the provider's responsibility; the CMA should defer diagnostic questions to the provider while ensuring the patient's concerns are communicated.
15. **C** – When a question asks for what to do "first," the best answer is usually the initial step that protects patient safety or begins appropriate assessment.
16. **B** – Asking for help so that infection-control standards are maintained balances workload with safety; skipping hand hygiene or leaving sharps is unsafe.
17. **B** – The Administrative domain includes tasks like reception, scheduling, records management, billing, and basic coding—not surgical or pharmaceutical tasks.
18. **B** – Using practice questions to find weak areas and then reviewing those topics is an efficient, targeted study strategy.
19. **C** – Missing scope-of-practice questions means you need to review that content and redo similar questions to strengthen understanding.
20. **B** – The exam expects behavior that follows policy, maintains accurate documentation, and stays within

scope; independent prescribing or skipping PPE is unsafe.

21. **B** – The CMA should finish essential clinical tasks and ensure the patient is safe before handling scheduling issues, reflecting proper prioritization.
22. **B** – The best response uses therapeutic communication and respects the patient's feelings, which aligns with exam expectations for professionalism.
23. **A** – Understanding how disease affects body systems is part of the General domain, which includes A&P and pathophysiology.
24. **C** – Knowing Clinical has the highest weight helps you allocate extra study time there while still covering General and Administrative domains.
25. **C** – Reviewing marked questions for misread words, safety issues, or scope violations is the best use of extra time and can improve your score.

Chapter 2

Professionalism, Legal/Ethical Practice, and Patient Rights

This chapter focuses on what it means to act like a health professional, not just a task-doer. You'll explore ethical principles, legal basics, confidentiality, consent, and key patient rights that shape day-to-day decisions. Many CMA exam questions in this area are short scenarios that test whether you choose the safest, most ethical option.

2.1 Defining Professionalism in Medical Assisting

PROFESSIONALISM IS more than wearing scrubs and showing up for work; it's about attitude, behavior, and reliability. Patients often judge the quality of the entire clinic based on their experience with you. The exam uses professionalism questions to see how you behave when things are stressful, busy, or emotionally charged.

- Consistent, dependable behavior and appearance
- Respectful communication with patients and coworkers

Being consistent and dependable means arriving on time, following the schedule, and completing tasks you accept. It includes keeping your workspace orderly and following through on messages, callbacks, and documentation. Professional appearance involves clean, appropriate clothing, good hygiene, and adherence to workplace dress codes. On the exam, answers that show responsibility and reliability—rather than excuses or shortcuts—usually reflect the professional choice.

Respectful communication means speaking to patients, providers, and coworkers in a calm, courteous way, even when you are frustrated. It includes avoiding gossip, sarcasm, or eye-rolling, and not discussing internal conflicts in front of patients. When two answers seem plausible, the professional one is usually the one that maintains dignity for everyone involved. The exam often rewards choices that de-escalate tension, protect relationships, and keep focus on patient care rather than personal drama.

2.2 Core Ethical Principles in Health Care

ETHICS GUIDES HOW YOU decide what is "the right thing" to do in difficult situations. You're not expected to be a philosopher, but you should recognize the main ethical principles that appear in the exam's scenarios. These principles shape how you balance patient wishes, safety, and fairness.

- Autonomy, beneficence, and nonmaleficence
- Justice and fidelity

Autonomy means respecting a patient's right to make decisions about their own care, even if you personally disagree. Beneficence is the duty to act in the patient's best interest, while nonmaleficence is the obligation to "do no harm." On exam questions, actions that force patients into procedures they do not understand or consent to typically violate autonomy and beneficence. Correct answers often involve providing information, answering questions, and supporting informed choices rather than pressuring patients.

Justice involves fairness—treating patients equitably regardless of background, income, or personal feelings. Fidelity means being faithful to your promises and responsibilities, such as keeping confidentiality and following through on commitments. In exam scenarios, justice is reflected when care is not withheld because of bias or inconvenience. Fidelity appears when you honor agreed-upon plans and do not mislead patients or colleagues. When in doubt, choose the answer that is fair, honest, and keeps trust intact.

2.3 Legal Basics: Negligence, Malpractice, and Liability

CMAS ARE NOT LAWYERS, but you need a basic understanding of legal concepts that appear when something goes wrong. Negligence and malpractice questions test whether you recognize risky behavior before it leads to harm. Knowing the legal landscape also reminds you why policies and documentation matter so much.

- Negligence and malpractice concepts
- Vicarious liability and the importance of following policy

Negligence occurs when someone fails to use reasonable care and a patient is harmed as a result. Malpractice is a form of professional negligence, usually involving a licensed provider failing to meet the standard of care. While CMAs are not typically sued alone, their actions can still become part of a malpractice case. On the exam, ignoring orders, skipping safety steps, or failing to report significant changes are red flags for negligence.

Vicarious liability means an employer or supervising provider can be held responsible for the actions of employees performed within the scope of employment. This is one reason policies and protocols are so detailed and why you must follow them closely. If a question shows a CMA ignoring policy "just this once," that answer is usually wrong. Correct choices involve following written procedures, clarifying unclear orders, and documenting what you did and when.

2.4 Confidentiality and Privacy (Including HIPAA Concepts)

CONFIDENTIALITY AND privacy are non-negotiable in health care. While the exam may not drill down into every technical detail of HIPAA, it will test whether you protect patient information in everyday situations. Many questions hinge on whether you recognize where private information is being exposed.

- Keeping patient information private in spoken and written form
- Handling records, screens, and conversations in public spaces

Keeping information private means only sharing it with people who are authorized and who need it to care for the patient. This includes staff who are part of the treatment team, certain insurers, or others named on a valid authorization. You should avoid discussing patients with friends or family members without permission, and never post information on social media. Exam questions often present a "casual conversation" that seems harmless but is actually a confidentiality violation.

Handling records correctly means being mindful of where screens face, where printed documents are left, and how conversations are conducted. You should log out or lock the computer when stepping away, and store charts or printed results in secure locations. In public spaces like waiting rooms, hallways, and elevators, you must avoid discussing specific patient details. On the exam, the best answer is usually the one that prevents unauthorized people from seeing or hearing protected information, even if it requires extra time or effort.

2.5 Consent, Informed Consent, and Implied Consent

CONSENT IS A PATIENT'S permission for care, and it has several forms the exam expects you to recognize. You won't be the one obtaining complex informed consent for major procedures, but you do need to understand what valid consent looks like. Questions often ask which action is appropriate when consent is unclear or missing.

- Basic and informed consent
- Implied consent in routine care situations

Basic consent is often verbal or implied and covers everyday procedures like taking vital signs or drawing blood, once the patient understands what you're doing. Informed consent is a more formal process, usually for significant procedures, where the provider explains risks, benefits, and alternatives. Your role often includes reinforcing information and checking that the patient understands, but not performing the full consent discussion. On the exam, any answer where you proceed with a major procedure without clear consent is likely incorrect.

Implied consent occurs when the patient's behavior indicates permission—for example, rolling up a sleeve when you explain that you need to take a blood pressure test. It does not apply to invasive or risky procedures that require explicit informed consent. If a patient refuses even a simple procedure, you must respect that decision and notify the provider. Exam questions in this area often reward answers that pause for clarification when a patient seems confused or hesitant, rather than pushing ahead.

2.6 Patient Rights and Responsibilities

PATIENTS HAVE SPECIFIC rights that protect their autonomy, dignity, and access to information. They also have responsibilities that help the healthcare team provide effective care. The exam checks whether you support these rights in your daily actions as a CMA.

- Key patient rights: information, privacy, and participation in decisions
- Patient responsibilities in the care partnership

Patients have the right to receive understandable information about their diagnosis, treatment options, and potential risks. They also have a right to privacy and to have their records kept confidential. Another key right is participation in decisions about their own care; they can accept or refuse treatments within legal limits. On exam questions, answers that respect the patient's right to ask questions, say "no," or request a second opinion usually align with these rights.

Patient responsibilities include giving accurate health information, following agreed-upon treatment plans as best they can, and communicating when they cannot comply. They are also responsible for asking questions when they do not understand instructions and for treating staff respectfully. While unmet responsibilities never justify violating patient rights, they do shape how the healthcare team responds. On the exam, you'll often see correct answers that encourage patients to engage actively in their care without blaming or shaming them.

2.7 Professional Boundaries and Workplace Harassment

PROFESSIONAL BOUNDARIES define appropriate limits in relationships with patients and coworkers. Crossing these lines can harm patients, damage trust, and create legal risk. The exam may use boundary or harassment scenarios to test whether you respond appropriately and seek help when needed.

- Maintaining clear boundaries with patients
- Recognizing and responding to harassment or inappropriate behavior

Maintaining boundaries means keeping the relationship focused on patient care rather than personal needs. This includes avoiding romantic or overly personal relationships with patients, not sharing excessive personal information, and not accepting large gifts or favors. Social media adds another layer; "friending" patients or messaging them privately about their care is usually inappropriate. On exam questions, the right answer typically involves redirecting the interaction back to care, or notifying a supervisor when boundaries are at risk.

Workplace harassment can come from patients, coworkers, or even supervisors. It may be sexual, verbal, or based on protected characteristics such as race or religion. You should know your facility's policy on reporting harassment and never be expected to tolerate abusive behavior. In exam scenarios, ignoring ongoing harassment is rarely the correct choice. More appropriate answers involve documenting incidents, following reporting procedures, and seeking support from appropriate leaders or human resources.

2.8 Cultural, Religious, and Individual Differences

PATIENTS BRING UNIQUE cultural, religious, and personal backgrounds into the exam room. Respecting these differences is both an ethical obligation and a practical necessity for effective care. The exam may present scenarios where you must choose a response that honors a patient's values while keeping them safe.

- Respecting cultural and religious practices in care
- Adapting communication and education to individual needs

Respecting cultural practices might involve adjusting scheduling or procedures to accommodate prayer times, dietary restrictions, or modesty concerns. Religious beliefs may influence whether a patient accepts certain treatments, such as blood products or specific procedures. You are not required to agree with every belief, but you must treat patients respectfully and help them understand their options. On the exam, answers that mock, ignore, or override a patient's beliefs without discussion are rarely correct.

Adapting communication involves considering language, literacy, and learning style. This may mean using interpreter services, providing written materials at an appropriate reading level, or using diagrams and models. Teach-back—asking patients to repeat instructions in their own words—is a powerful tool the exam often rewards. When two answers seem reasonable, the better one usually checks for understanding and respects the patient's background rather than delivering a one-size-fits-all explanation.

2.9 Documentation, Errors, and Incident Reporting

DOCUMENTATION IS YOUR written record of what happened and when, and it has legal and clinical importance. Errors and incidents need to be handled transparently and according to policy. The exam tests whether you know how to document correctly and what to do when something goes wrong.

- Objective, accurate documentation practices
- Reporting errors and incidents according to policy

Objective documentation means charting facts rather than opinions. You record what you see, hear, and do, along with patient responses, using clear, professional language. You avoid judgmental terms and never alter records to hide mistakes. If you need to correct an entry, you follow facility procedures, such as adding an addendum or electronic correction with your name, date, and reason. On the exam, answers that involve erasing, backdating, or deleting information are almost always wrong.

When an error or incident occurs—such as a medication mistake, fall, or needle-stick—you must report it promptly. This typically involves notifying the appropriate provider or supervisor and completing an incident report that is separate from the medical record. The incident report should be factual and detailed but not used to assign blame. Exam questions generally favor answers that prioritize patient safety, immediate assessment, and honest reporting rather than hiding or minimizing the event.

2.10 Handling Difficult Situations and Ethical Dilemmas

HEALTHCARE CAN INVOLVE emotionally charged, complex situations where there is no perfect answer. The CMA exam may present ethical dilemmas to see if you recognize your role and respond appropriately. You're not expected to solve every ethical problem alone, but you should know how to act safely and escalate concerns.

- Recognizing when a situation is beyond your role
- Seeking guidance from supervisors, ethics resources, or the provider

Some situations—such as family conflicts over end-of-life care or disagreements about risky procedures—are beyond the CMA's authority to resolve. Your job is to provide accurate information within your scope, support the patient respectfully, and alert the provider or nurse to concerns. Trying to give independent advice on complex ethical or medical issues is not appropriate. On the exam, answers that keep you within scope and bring the issue to the right person are usually correct.

Seeking guidance may involve talking to your immediate supervisor, the provider responsible for the patient, or institutional resources such as an ethics committee. You might also consult written policies or professional guidelines. The exam favors options where you acknowledge uncertainty and ask for help rather than guessing. Ethical practice is not about having all the answers; it is about recognizing limits and making sure the patient's rights and safety remain at the center of decisions.

Practice Questions – Chapter 2 (25 Questions)

THESE QUESTIONS FOCUS on Chapter 2 topics: professionalism, ethics, legal basics, confidentiality, consent, patient rights, boundaries, cultural issues, documentation, and handling dilemmas.

1. A CMA arrives late several times a week and often leaves tasks unfinished for the next shift. This behavior primarily violates which aspect of professionalism?
   A. Respectful communication
   B. Dependability and reliability
   C. Dress code policy
   D. Scope of practice
2. A patient becomes upset and speaks harshly to the CMA about a delay. What is the **most professional** response?
   A. "If you don't calm down, you can leave."
   B. "We're busy; you'll just have to wait."
   C. "I understand this is frustrating. I'll check on your wait time and let you know what to expect."
   D. "You're not the only patient here."
3. A patient refuses a flu vaccine after the CMA explains the benefits. Which ethical principle is most directly involved in respecting this decision?
   A. Justice
   B. Autonomy
   C. Fidelity
   D. Nonmaleficence
4. A provider asks a CMA to perform a procedure the CMA has never been trained to do. What is the **best** action?
   A. Attempt the procedure to avoid upsetting the provider
   B. Ask a coworker to do it without telling the provider
   C. Tell the provider you have not been trained and request clarification or training
   D. Refuse all future tasks from that provider
5. A CMA fails to secure the side rails on an exam table, and a patient falls and is injured. This situation best illustrates:
   A. Patient autonomy
   B. Standard of care
   C. Negligence
   D. Beneficence
6. Which scenario is the **clearest violation** of patient confidentiality?
   A. Calling a patient's name in the waiting room
   B. Reviewing a chart at the nurses' station
   C. Discussing a patient's diagnosis with a friend over lunch
   D. Verifying a patient's date of birth during check-in
7. A patient's spouse calls asking for lab results, stating, "We share everything." The CMA should:
   A. Give the results because spouses always have the right to know
   B. Refuse to give any information to anyone over the phone
   C. Verify whether a valid authorization exists before releasing information
   D. Read the results but avoid explaining them
8. Which best describes **informed consent**?
   A. The patient quietly lets the CMA proceed without asking questions
   B. The provider explains the procedure, risks, benefits, and alternatives, and the patient agrees
   C. The CMA signs the consent form for the patient

D. The patient nods when the CMA walks in

9. A patient rolls up a sleeve and extends their arm after the CMA explains that they will take a blood pressure. This is an example of:
   A. Implied consent
   B. Informed consent
   C. Coerced consent
   D. No consent
10. A patient requests copies of their medical record. How should the CMA respond?
   A. "You are not allowed to see your own record."
   B. "You can have access according to our facility's policies and procedures."
   C. "We only release records to insurance companies."
   D. "You may see your record only if the provider approves the content."
11. A CMA receives an expensive gift card from a patient after a procedure. What is the **most appropriate** response?
   A. Accept the gift and say nothing
   B. Accept the gift and ask for a larger one next time
   C. Thank the patient but explain that clinic policy does not allow accepting expensive gifts
   D. Sell the gift card and share the money with coworkers
12. A coworker makes repeated inappropriate comments about a CMA's appearance after being asked to stop. What should the CMA do next?
   A. Ignore it and hope it stops
   B. Respond with equally inappropriate comments
   C. Document the behavior and follow workplace procedures for reporting harassment
   D. Quit immediately without telling anyone why
13. A patient's religious beliefs prohibit blood transfusions. The CMA should:
   A. Try to convince the patient to change their beliefs
   B. Mock the belief in front of other staff
   C. Respect the belief and notify the provider so alternatives can be discussed
   D. Administer blood products secretly for the patient's own good
14. During patient education, the CMA notices the patient looks confused and is not asking questions. What is the **best** next step?
   A. Assume the patient understands and move on
   B. Speak more quickly to save time
   C. Ask the patient to repeat the instructions in their own words (teach-back)
   D. Tell the patient to read the brochure at home
15. Which documentation entry is most appropriate?
   A. "The patient is lazy and refuses to follow instructions."
   B. "Patients are stupid about their disease."
   C. "Patient states, 'I don't understand how to use this inhaler.' Education provided and demonstration practice."
   D. "The patient is annoying and noncompliant."
16. After accidentally giving a patient the wrong dose of medication, the CMA's **first priority** is to:
   A. Hide the error to avoid punishment
   B. Tell coworkers not to mention it

C. Assess the patient's condition and notify the provider immediately
D. Leave at the end of the shift and hope the patient is fine

17. An incident report should:
A. Be used to punish staff
B. Include objective facts about what happened, without blaming language
C. Be placed in the patient's medical record
D. Be written in casual, informal language
18. A patient is upset because they feel they were treated unfairly compared with other patients. Which ethical principle is most involved?
A. Autonomy
B. Justice
C. Fidelity
D. Nonmaleficence
19. A patient angrily states, "I'm not going to follow this diet; it's too hard." What is the **most appropriate** CMA response?
A. "Then don't complain when you get sicker."
B. "You have to follow it exactly or it's pointless."
C. "It sounds overwhelming. Let's talk about what parts feel hardest and what you can realistically try."
D. "Your choices are your problem, not mine."
20. A CMA is unsure whether a situation involves reportable abuse. What should they do?
A. Decide on their own that it probably isn't abuse
B. Ignore the concerns and continue working
C. Discuss the observations with the provider or supervisor and follow reporting policy
D. Ask other patients if they think it is abuse
21. On the exam, a scenario describes a complex ethical conflict between a family and a provider. The CMA should generally:
A. Take sides with whichever party seems more reasonable
B. Offer personal opinions about what the family should decide
C. Stay within scope, support communication, and direct concerns to the provider
D. Make the final decision to resolve the conflict
22. Which action best demonstrates **fidelity**?
A. Treating all patients fairly
B. Keeping promises, such as returning calls when you say you will
C. Avoiding harm to patients
D. Respecting patient choices
23. A CMA posts a funny but de-identified story about a clinic incident on social media. No names are used. This action is:
A. Always acceptable because no names were mentioned
B. Potentially problematic if details could identify the patient or clinic
C. Encouraged for team morale
D. Required for transparency
24. A patient with limited English proficiency nods but seems confused when given instructions in English. The **best** action is to:
A. Continue in English because nodding means understanding

B. Speak louder and slower in English
C. Use a qualified medical interpreter and verify understanding with teach-back
D. Ask a child in the room to translate

25. A CMA notices they feel personally irritated by a particular patient and finds themselves wanting to rush through the visit. What should they do?
A. Let their feelings guide how they treat the patient
B. Recognize the feeling, refocus on professional behavior, and provide the same standard of care
C. Tell the patient they are difficult
D. Ask to never care for that patient again without explanation

Answer Key – Chapter 2 (with Justifications)

1. **B** – Repeated lateness and leaving tasks unfinished show a lack of dependability and reliability, which is a core part of professionalism.
2. **C** – Acknowledging the patient's frustration and checking on their wait time is professional, empathetic, and focused on problem-solving.
3. **B** – Autonomy is the patient's right to make decisions about their own care, including refusing a recommended vaccine.
4. **C** – The CMA must not perform tasks for which they have not been trained; the correct action is to inform the provider and request training or clarification.
5. **C** – Failing to secure side rails, leading to patient injury, is an example of negligence—failure to use reasonable care resulting in harm.
6. **C** – Discussing a patient's diagnosis with a friend is a clear breach of confidentiality; the other actions are normal aspects of patient care.
7. **C** – The CMA must verify that appropriate authorization exists before releasing information, even to a spouse.
8. **B** – Informed consent requires an explanation of the procedure, risks, benefits, and alternatives, followed by the patient's agreement.
9. **A** – The patient's action of rolling up a sleeve after explanation is implied consent for a routine, low-risk procedure.
10. **B** – Patients have a right to access their own records according to facility policies and legal requirements.
11. **C** – Politely declining an expensive gift and referencing clinic policy maintains professional boundaries and avoids conflicts of interest.
12. **C** – Ongoing inappropriate comments should be documented and reported according to workplace harassment procedures; ignoring them is not adequate.
13. **C** – Respecting the patient's beliefs and notifying the provider allows discussion of alternatives without violating autonomy or religious freedom.
14. **C** – Using teach-back helps ensure the patient truly understands instructions and is a best practice for patient education.
15. **C** – This entry is objective, quotes the patient directly, and documents education provided, avoiding judgmental language.
16. **C** – After an error, the immediate priority is patient safety: assess the patient and notify the provider; hiding the error is unethical and unsafe.
17. **B** – Incident reports should contain objective facts about what happened, not blame or emotional language,

and are not placed in the medical record.

18. **B** – Justice is the ethical principle related to fairness and equal treatment, which is at issue when a patient feels treated unfairly.
19. **C** – This response acknowledges difficulty, uses therapeutic communication, and seeks a realistic plan instead of blaming or shaming.
20. **C** – When unsure about possible abuse, the CMA should discuss observations with a provider or supervisor and follow the facility's reporting policy.
21. **C** – In complex ethical conflicts, the CMA should stay within scope, facilitate communication, and refer concerns to the provider rather than making decisions.
22. **B** – Fidelity involves keeping promises and being faithful to commitments, such as returning calls when promised.
23. **B** – Even without names, details can sometimes identify patients or facilities, making social media posts potentially problematic and unprofessional.
24. **C** – Using a qualified medical interpreter and verifying understanding with teach-back best ensures accurate, safe communication for a limited-English patient.
25. **B** – Recognizing personal feelings and consciously refocusing on professional behavior ensures that all patients receive the same standard of care.

Chapter 3

Communication, Interpersonal Skills, and Cultural Competence

Communication is where a medical assistant either builds trust or accidentally breaks it. This chapter focuses on how you talk with patients, families, coworkers, and providers—and how you adapt your style to different situations and cultures. Many CMA exam questions test these "soft skills" because they're critical for safety, patient satisfaction, and teamwork.

3.1 Foundations of Therapeutic Communication

THERAPEUTIC COMMUNICATION is intentional communication that supports the patient's emotional and psychological needs while exchanging information. It goes beyond casual conversation and focuses on listening, empathy, and clarity. The exam uses these concepts to see whether you help or hinder patients when they're stressed or confused.

- Active listening and presence
- Empathy and nonjudgmental attitude

Active listening means giving the patient your full attention, rather than thinking about your next task while they speak. It includes maintaining appropriate eye contact, nodding, and using short prompts like "go on" or "I see" to encourage them to continue. You also avoid interrupting unless necessary, and you reflect key ideas back to confirm understanding. On the exam, answers that show active listening usually involve letting the patient speak, checking understanding, and avoiding distractions or multitasking mid-conversation.

Empathy involves trying to understand what the patient feels and showing that you care, without judging or taking over their experience. A nonjudgmental attitude means you don't criticize choices, lifestyles, or emotions, even if you don't personally agree with them. Instead, you focus on supporting the patient and helping them move toward better health. In exam scenarios, responses that criticize, shame, or minimize the patient's feelings are almost always wrong. The correct answers recognize emotions, validate them, and keep the door open for more discussion.

3.2 Verbal Communication Techniques

VERBAL COMMUNICATION is not just what you say, but how you say it. The CMA is expected to use clear, simple language and to choose words that help, not confuse. The exam tests whether you can adapt your spoken communication to the patient's needs and the situation.

- Using plain language and avoiding jargon
- Asking open-ended vs. closed-ended questions

Using plain language means replacing complex medical terms with words patients are likely to understand, or clearly explaining medical terms when they are necessary. You might say "high blood pressure" instead of "hypertension," or "heart doctor" instead of "cardiologist" when appropriate. Tone of voice, speed, and volume also matter; speaking too quickly or too softly can reduce understanding. On the exam, answers that prioritize simplicity, clarity, and calm tone tend to be better choices than those that rely on technical jargon to sound impressive.

Open-ended questions invite longer responses and help you gather more information, such as "Can you tell me more about your pain?" Closed-ended questions can be answered with a simple "yes" or "no," and are useful when you need specific details like "Did the pain start today?" Effective communication usually uses both types, but relies more on open-ended questions early in an assessment. Exam questions often reward answers that start with open-ended questions to understand the problem, then use closed-ended questions to clarify details.

3.3 Nonverbal Communication and Professional Body Language

NONVERBAL COMMUNICATION includes facial expressions, posture, gestures, and physical distance. Patients pick up on these signals even when you're not speaking. The exam may give you clues about body language to see if you notice what message is being sent.

- Body language that builds trust
- Nonverbal cues that can harm communication

Body language that builds trust includes facing the patient, maintaining an open posture, and sitting or standing at a comfortable distance. You avoid crossing your arms, checking your watch, or looking at your phone while they talk. A calm facial expression and nodding can show that you are engaged and not rushing them. Exam questions often describe a CMA who sits down, looks at the patient, and listens calmly—this is usually the positive model.

Nonverbal cues that harm communication include eye-rolling, sighing, tapping your foot, frowning, or looking impatient. Even if your words are polite, these signals can make patients feel judged, dismissed, or unwelcome. Turning away from the patient or working on the computer without looking up can also send the message that you are not listening. On the exam, these negative cues are often included as red flags that suggest a wrong answer, even if the spoken words in the option sound okay.

3.4 Communication Across the Lifespan

DIFFERENT AGE GROUPS have different needs, abilities, and preferences when it comes to communication. A message that works for an adult may be confusing or frightening to a child or not loud and clear enough for an older adult. The exam tests whether you tailor your approach based on the patient's stage of life.

- Communicating with children and adolescents
- Communicating with older adults

When communicating with children, you typically use simple words, a calm tone, and concrete examples. You might demonstrate a procedure on a doll or show equipment before using it. With younger children, involving a parent or caregiver is essential, while still speaking directly to the child at their level. For adolescents, you may need to balance privacy and parental involvement, especially on sensitive topics. Exam answers that respect developmental level—rather than talking to a child like an adult or ignoring the adolescent's voice—are usually correct.

Older adults may have hearing, vision, or cognitive changes that affect how they receive information. Speaking clearly, facing the patient so they can see your lips, and minimizing background noise can help. You may need to provide written instructions in large print or repeat key points calmly. It's important not to assume that all older adults are confused or incapable; many are fully independent and sharp. On the exam, answers that show patience, respect, and adapted techniques without being patronizing tend to be favored.

3.5 Managing Difficult Emotions and Challenging Behaviors

PATIENTS SOMETIMES express fear, anger, sadness, or frustration—and these emotions can be directed at you, even when you're not the cause. Challenging behaviors can include yelling, refusing treatments, or withdrawing completely. The exam measures whether you respond in a way that is safe, professional, and helpful.

- Responding to anger or frustration
- Supporting anxious, fearful, or tearful patients

When patients are angry or frustrated, your job is to stay calm and avoid taking it personally. You might acknowledge their feelings—"I can see this is really upsetting"—and explain what you can do to help. Setting respectful boundaries is also important, such as reminding a patient that abusive language is not acceptable while still offering assistance. On exam questions, escalating the conflict, arguing, or threatening the patient is almost always the wrong choice. Remaining calm and focused on solutions points to the best answer.

Anxious or fearful patients often need extra reassurance and clear explanations. You can help by describing what will happen step by step, allowing time for questions, and normalizing feelings like nervousness. Sometimes simple measures—slower speech, a gentler tone, or offering to pause if they feel overwhelmed—make a big difference. Tearful patients may need tissues, a moment of silence, or a chance to talk about what worries them. Exam scenarios typically reward answers that validate emotions and provide support rather than minimizing or ignoring the distress.

3.6 Communication Within the Healthcare Team

COMMUNICATION IS NOT just between you and patients; it also occurs within the healthcare team. Miscommunication between staff can lead to errors, delays, and frustration. The exam evaluates whether you share information accurately, respectfully, and through proper channels.

- Giving concise, accurate reports and messages
- Respectful collaboration and conflict resolution

Giving effective reports means providing the right information in a clear, organized way. You might use a structured format like identifying the patient, stating the problem, giving relevant facts, and explaining what you need from the provider or nurse. Avoiding vague phrases like "they look bad" and instead using vital signs or specific observations helps others understand the situation quickly. On exam questions, correct answers often show the CMA giving clear, concise, and factual information rather than rambling or leaving out key details.

Respectful collaboration means working with coworkers as partners, not rivals. Disagreements are inevitable, but how you handle them is what matters. You should address concerns privately when possible, focus on the issue rather than attacking the person, and be open to feedback. If a conflict affects patient care, involving a supervisor may be appropriate. The exam usually favors responses that protect teamwork and patient safety instead of gossip, public arguments, or blaming.

3.7 Cultural Competence and Health Literacy

CULTURAL COMPETENCE means being aware of, respectful toward, and responsive to cultural differences in health beliefs and practices. Health literacy refers to a patient's ability to obtain, understand, and use health information. The exam uses these concepts to test whether you can adapt education and communication to the individual patient.

- Respecting cultural differences in beliefs and practices
- Adjusting explanations for varying health literacy levels

Respecting cultural differences might involve understanding that some patients prefer family involvement in decisions, while others value privacy and independence. Some cultures may use traditional remedies alongside medical care, or have beliefs about illness that differ from biomedical explanations. You don't need to know every tradition, but you should ask respectful questions and avoid assumptions. On the exam, answers that dismiss or mock cultural beliefs are usually incorrect; the better responses seek understanding and find safe ways to integrate care.

Health literacy affects whether a patient can follow instructions, take medications correctly, and recognize warning signs. You should avoid overloading patients with complex information, especially if they seem overwhelmed. Using short sentences, everyday words, pictures, and teach-back can make instructions more understandable. Patients may feel embarrassed to admit they don't understand, so exam answers often reward proactive checks for comprehension rather than "Do you understand?" which often leads to a forced "yes."

3.8 Telephone and Electronic Communication

MUCH OF A CMA'S COMMUNICATION happens through phones, patient portals, and electronic messages. These methods require clarity, confidentiality, and adherence to protocols. The exam checks whether you handle calls and electronic communication safely and professionally.

- Handling patient phone calls appropriately
- Using electronic communication and patient portals safely

When handling calls, you should identify yourself and your role, verify the patient's identity using facility-approved identifiers, and use a structured method for taking messages. You never give diagnostic opinions or change treatment plans over the phone on your own. Instead, you document the call and route it to the appropriate provider or nurse when needed. On exam questions, guessing at diagnoses or giving medication advice outside of protocol is usually wrong; the correct answer follows telephone triage policies.

Electronic communication, such as secure messaging or portals, requires careful attention to privacy and documentation. You must avoid sending health information through unsecured channels and follow facility rules for responding to messages. Written messages should be clear, professional, and free of slang or emotional language. The exam often favors answers that use official, secure systems over personal email or texting, and that document important patient communications in the record.

3.9 Overcoming Communication Barriers

BARRIERS TO COMMUNICATION can include language differences, sensory impairments, cognitive limitations, and environmental distractions. As a CMA, you're expected to recognize these barriers and take steps to reduce them. The exam tests whether you choose strategies that improve understanding and safety.

- Language barriers and interpreter use

- Sensory and cognitive barriers

Language barriers require more than just speaking louder or slower. For patients with limited English proficiency, the best practice is to use a qualified medical interpreter rather than family members, especially children. You should still address the patient directly, not the interpreter, and allow extra time for the conversation. On the exam, using untrained interpreters or relying on gestures and guessing is less safe; using professional interpreter services and verifying understanding is typically the correct choice.

Sensory barriers include hearing or vision problems, while cognitive barriers may involve memory issues, confusion, or developmental conditions. For hearing impairments, facing the patient, speaking clearly, and reducing background noise can help. For vision impairments, verbal explanations and tactile cues may be more important than printed materials. When cognitive issues are present, shorter sentences, repetition, and involving caregivers can improve understanding. Exam questions often reward answers that adapt communication to the barrier rather than treating all patients the same way.

3.10 De-escalation and Professional Self-Control

SOMETIMES SITUATIONS become heated, and the CMA must help de-escalate them. Professional self-control means managing your own reactions so you can respond thoughtfully rather than emotionally. The exam frequently presents tense scenarios to see if you can calm things down instead of making them worse.

- Techniques for de-escalating tense interactions
- Managing your own emotions and stress

De-escalation techniques include using a calm tone, maintaining a non-threatening posture, and giving the person space when possible. You may acknowledge their feelings—"I can see you're very upset"—and set limits calmly, such as stating that abusive language is not acceptable. Offering specific options ("We can do X now, or Y later") can help people feel less trapped. On the exam, yelling back, making threats, or walking away abruptly are usually wrong; answers that focus on calm, safety, and clear boundaries are preferred.

Managing your own emotions involves recognizing when you are frustrated, anxious, or overwhelmed and taking steps to stay professional. This might mean pausing to take a breath, asking for brief backup from a coworker, or debriefing with a supervisor after a difficult encounter. Self-care outside of work—sleep, nutrition, stress management—also affects how well you communicate. Exam scenarios will favor options where you keep your composure and avoid reacting impulsively, even when others are rude or angry.

Practice Questions – Chapter 3 (25 Questions)

THESE QUESTIONS FOCUS on Chapter 3 content: therapeutic communication, verbal/nonverbal skills, lifespan differences, managing emotions, team communication, cultural competence, health literacy, phone/electronic communication, barriers, and de-escalation.

1. A patient says, "I'm really scared about this test. I don't know what's going to happen." Which response best demonstrates **therapeutic communication**?
   A. "You'll be fine. It's not a big deal."
   B. "There's nothing to be scared of."

C. "It sounds like you're feeling pretty anxious. Let's talk about what the test involves and what you can expect."
D. "You agreed to the test, so you shouldn't be scared now."

2. Which behavior shows **active listening**?
A. Typing on the computer while the patient talks and not looking up
B. Interrupting to tell the patient about your own experience
C. Making eye contact, nodding, and reflecting key points back to the patient
D. Checking your watch frequently during the conversation
3. Which question is **open-ended** and most helpful for beginning an assessment?
A. "Does it hurt?"
B. "Is your pain a 10 out of 10?"
C. "When did the pain start?"
D. "Can you tell me in your own words what brought you in today?"
4. A patient looks down and speaks in a very soft voice when answering questions. What is the **best** initial response from the CMA?
A. "Speak up; I can't hear you."
B. "You need to look at me when you talk."
C. Use a gentle tone, sit at eye level, and ask, "I notice you seem a little uncomfortable. Would you like to talk about what's worrying you?"
D. Ignore it and move on quickly
5. Which nonverbal behavior is most likely to make a patient feel **judged or dismissed**?
A. Nodding and leaning slightly forward
B. Maintaining neutral facial expression
C. Rolling your eyes and sighing
D. Sitting at eye level
6. When communicating with a 6-year-old about a blood draw, the CMA should:
A. Use detailed anatomical terms to sound professional
B. Explain simply, possibly using a doll or visual, and allow questions
C. Avoid explaining anything to prevent fear
D. Only talk to the parent and ignore the child
7. An older adult patient has mild hearing loss. Which strategy is most appropriate?
A. Shouting loudly in one ear
B. Facing the patient, speaking clearly, and reducing background noise
C. Speaking very quickly to get through instructions
D. Giving instructions only in writing
8. A patient is yelling about wait times at the front desk. What is the **most appropriate** CMA response?
A. Yell back to show you're not intimidated
B. Tell them they can leave if they don't like it
C. Calmly acknowledge their frustration and explain what you can do to check on delays
D. Ignore them until they stop yelling
9. A coworker gives a report that is long and unfocused, leaving out vital signs. What communication principle is most important here?
A. The report should be emotional and detailed
B. The report should be concise, organized, and include key clinical facts

C. The report should be humorous to keep morale high
D. The report should avoid mentioning patient problems

10. A patient from a different cultural background uses traditional remedies along with prescribed medications. What is the **best** CMA response?
A. "Those remedies are useless; stop them immediately."
B. "That's interesting. Can you tell me more about what you're using so I can let the provider know?"
C. "We don't allow any cultural practices here."
D. "As long as you feel better, we don't need to know about them."

11. A patient seems overwhelmed by discharge instructions. Which approach best supports **low health literacy**?
A. Speaking more quickly to get through everything
B. Using short sentences, simple words, and checking understanding with teach-back
C. Giving a thick stack of written information and leaving
D. Asking, "Do you understand?" and accepting "yes" without further questions

12. A patient with limited English proficiency comes alone to the clinic. The **best** communication strategy is to:
A. Ask a child in the waiting room to interpret
B. Use gestures instead of words
C. Use a qualified medical interpreter and speak directly to the patient
D. Refuse to see the patient until they bring an English-speaking family member

13. The CMA answers a phone call from a patient complaining of chest pain at rest. What is the **most appropriate** response?
A. Tell the patient to wait and see if it improves
B. Provide detailed medical advice from memory
C. Instruct the patient to call emergency services immediately and notify the provider according to protocol
D. Schedule the next available appointment in several days

14. When using the phone for routine questions, the CMA should:
A. Avoid documenting the call
B. Identify themselves and verify the patient's identity using approved identifiers
C. Share details freely with anyone who says they are family
D. Use personal opinions to respond

15. Which electronic communication practice is **most appropriate**?
A. Sending lab results to a patient via personal email without encryption
B. Using secure patient portal messaging according to facility policy
C. Texting results from your personal phone for convenience
D. Posting general patient information in a group chat

16. A patient begins to cry during a visit and says, "I'm just so tired of dealing with this." What is the **best** CMA response?
A. "You need to be stronger."
B. "This isn't that bad compared to other patients."
C. "It sounds like this has been really exhausting for you. Would you like to talk more about how it's affecting you?"
D. "You shouldn't cry in a doctor's office."

17. A patient stares at the floor and doesn't answer questions about medication use. What is the best first step?
A. Accuse the patient of hiding information
B. Use a gentle, nonjudgmental question like, "Many people sometimes miss doses. How often do you think

that happens for you?"
C. Tell the patient the provider will be angry
D. Move on without asking again

18. A CMA is feeling stressed and rushed but must speak with an anxious patient. The **best** approach is to:
A. Bring your stress into the conversation to move faster
B. Take a brief moment to breathe and refocus, then communicate calmly
C. Tell the patient you're too busy to talk
D. Walk away until you feel better, without explanation

19. A patient with dementia repeatedly asks the same question about an upcoming test. The most appropriate response is to:
A. Become irritated and tell them to stop asking
B. Answer once and ignore all future repetitions
C. Respond patiently, using simple explanations and reassurance each time
D. Tell them the test was canceled even if it was not

20. A CMA notices a coworker speaking harshly and rolling their eyes at a confused patient. The CMA's **best** initial action is to:
A. Join in to avoid conflict
B. Ignore the behavior to stay out of it
C. Speak with the coworker privately, expressing concern about how it might affect the patient, and seek guidance if it continues
D. Publicly criticize the coworker in front of patients

21. During a team conflict about responsibilities, the CMA should:
A. Blame others to avoid taking responsibility
B. Focus on personal grievances only
C. Communicate concerns respectfully, focus on patient care, and be open to compromise
D. Refuse to participate in any discussion

22. A patient comes from a culture where the family makes most medical decisions. The **best** approach is to:
A. Refuse to talk to family members at all
B. Insist the patient decide alone regardless of their preference
C. Ask the patient how they prefer decisions to be made and involve family as appropriate with the patient's permission
D. Allow family to make all decisions without asking the patient

23. Which of the following is a **barrier** that might require an adapted communication strategy?
A. The clinic being open on weekends
B. The patient wearing a jacket
C. The patient having significant hearing loss
D. The CMA using a computer

24. A patient becomes increasingly agitated, pacing and raising their voice. What is the **best** de-escalation step?
A. Move closer and speak loudly to show control
B. Use a calm tone, maintain a safe distance, and set clear limits about behavior
C. Make fun of the patient to distract them
D. Order the patient to sit down immediately

25. A CMA is giving discharge instructions and notices the patient nods but looks confused. What should the CMA do?

A. Assume the nodding means understanding and continue
B. Ask the patient to repeat the instructions in their own words and clarify as needed
C. Simply hand over written instructions and leave
D. Tell the patient to call back if there are problems, without further explanation

Answer Key – Chapter 3 (with Justifications)

1. **C** – This response acknowledges the patient's anxiety and offers clear information, which is the essence of therapeutic communication.
2. **C** – Active listening involves eye contact, nodding, and reflecting key points back, showing full engagement with the patient.
3. **D** – "Can you tell me in your own words what brought you in today?" is open-ended and invites a full description of the issue.
4. **C** – Sitting at eye level and gently exploring the patient's discomfort uses therapeutic communication instead of demanding or ignoring.
5. **C** – Eye-rolling and sighing are negative nonverbal cues that make patients feel judged or dismissed.
6. **B** – Simple explanations, possibly with a doll or visual, are appropriate for a young child and help reduce fear.
7. **B** – Facing the patient, speaking clearly, and minimizing noise supports communication with someone who has hearing loss.
8. **C** – Acknowledging frustration and checking on delays is professional and de-escalates tension rather than escalating it.
9. **B** – Reports should be concise, organized, and include essential clinical facts like vital signs to support safe care.
10. **B** – Asking respectfully about traditional remedies and informing the provider shows cultural sensitivity and protects safety.
11. **B** – Short sentences, simple words, and teach-back are key strategies for patients with low health literacy.
12. **C** – Using a qualified medical interpreter and addressing the patient directly is the safest and most professional approach.
13. **C** – Chest pain at rest may be an emergency; instructing the patient to call emergency services and notifying the provider follows safe protocols.
14. **B** – Identifying yourself and verifying the patient's identity with approved identifiers is essential for safe phone communication.
15. **B** – Secure patient portal messaging follows privacy rules and facility policy, unlike personal email or texting.
16. **C** – This response acknowledges the patient's exhaustion and invites further discussion, consistent with therapeutic communication.
17. **B** – A nonjudgmental, normalizing question about missed doses encourages honest communication without shaming.
18. **B** – Taking a brief moment to refocus and then communicating calmly helps prevent your stress from harming patient communication.
19. **C** – Responding patiently, with simple explanations and reassurance, is appropriate when dementia causes repeated questions.
20. **C** – Addressing the behavior privately and seeking guidance if needed supports professionalism and patient respect.
21. **C** – Respectful discussion focused on patient care and willingness to compromise are hallmarks of effective

team communication.

22. **C** – Asking the patient about their preferences and involving family with permission respects autonomy and culture.
23. **C** – Significant hearing loss is a communication barrier that requires adaptation (e.g., clearer speech, reduced noise).
24. **B** – A calm tone, safe distance, and clear behavioral limits are key de-escalation strategies.
25. **B** – Teach-back—asking the patient to repeat instructions—confirms understanding and allows for clarification where needed.

Chapter 4

Infection Control, Asepsis, and Safety

Infection control is one of the most heavily tested parts of the Clinical domain because it affects every patient, every day. As a CMA, you are often the first and last person to touch equipment, surfaces, and patients during a visit. This chapter focuses on the principles, procedures, and safety practices that keep both patients and staff safe from infection.

4.1 Chain of Infection and Key Principles

INFECTIONS DON'T JUST "appear"; they follow a predictable pattern called the chain of infection. Understanding each link in the chain helps you see where your actions can stop an infection from spreading. The exam often expects you to recognize which part of the chain you are interrupting with a particular measure.

- Links in the chain of infection
- Breaking the chain through targeted interventions

The chain of infection includes an infectious agent, a reservoir, a portal of exit, a mode of transmission, a portal of entry, and a susceptible host. Each step describes how germs move from one place to another and eventually cause disease. For example, a reservoir may be a person, surface, or piece of equipment that harbors microorganisms. On exam questions, recognizing which link is involved helps you understand why certain precautions (like cleaning a surface or covering a cough) matter.

Breaking the chain means applying specific interventions that block one or more links. Hand hygiene, cleaning equipment, using PPE, and vaccinating susceptible hosts are all ways to interrupt this process. Even something as simple as placing a mask on a coughing patient can reduce spread by blocking the portal of exit and mode of transmission. The exam tends to reward answers that clearly interrupt the chain in a realistic way, rather than vague or ineffective actions.

4.2 Standard Precautions and Hand Hygiene

STANDARD PRECAUTIONS are the foundation of infection control and apply to all patients, regardless of diagnosis. Hand hygiene is the most important single action you can take to prevent the spread of infection. The exam repeatedly tests whether you follow these basics even when the scenario pressures you to rush.

- Core components of Standard Precautions
- Proper hand hygiene technique and indications

Standard precautions include treating all blood and certain body fluids as potentially infectious and using barriers like gloves, masks, and gowns when exposure is possible. They also involve safe injection practices, respiratory hygiene, and appropriate handling of equipment and laundry. You are expected to use Standard Precautions for every patient, not just those who are visibly ill. On the exam, answers that suggest skipping these precautions because a patient "looks healthy" are almost always incorrect.

Proper hand hygiene can involve either alcohol-based hand rub or soap and water, depending on the situation. You should perform hand hygiene before and after contact with each patient, after removing gloves, after touching bodily fluids or contaminated surfaces, and before performing clean or invasive procedures. Soap and water are preferred when hands are visibly soiled or after contact with certain organisms like Clostridioides difficile. Questions often ask when hand hygiene is required; the safest answers typically err on the side of "wash more, not less."

4.3 Transmission-Based Precautions

WHILE STANDARD PRECAUTIONS apply to everyone, some patients require extra steps known as transmission-based precautions. These are tailored to how specific organisms spread. The CMA must recognize basic categories and what they mean in practice.

- Contact, droplet, and airborne precautions
- Patient placement and PPE selection

Contact precautions are used for infections spread by direct touch or contaminated surfaces, such as some skin infections or gastrointestinal illnesses. Droplet precautions address infections that spread in large respiratory droplets, like certain types of flu. Airborne precautions are for organisms that can travel on smaller particles over longer distances, such as tuberculosis. On the exam, recognizing the difference helps you pick appropriate measures, like gowns and gloves for contact or masks for droplet and airborne situations.

Patient placement involves choosing where and how a patient should be housed or seated, especially in waiting areas or shared rooms. For higher-risk cases, this may mean a private room or specific airflow controls for airborne diseases. PPE selection must match the type of precaution—gloves and gowns for contact, surgical masks for droplets, and specialized respirators for airborne, where required and within scope. Exam questions often present a scenario with cough, rash, or diarrhea and expect you to choose both correct PPE and safe placement.

4.4 Medical Asepsis: Cleaning, Disinfection, and Environmental Control

MEDICAL ASEPSIS IS the reduction of microorganisms to a safe level in everyday clinical settings. It includes cleaning and disinfecting surfaces, equipment, and the environment. The CMA plays a major role in implementing these practices correctly.

- Levels of decontamination: cleaning, disinfection, and sterilization
- Environmental cleaning and workflow in the outpatient setting

Cleaning removes visible dirt and organic material from surfaces and equipment, often with soap and water. Disinfection goes further by using chemical agents to reduce or eliminate many microorganisms, though not necessarily all spores. Sterilization, which completely destroys all forms of microbial life, is reserved for critical instruments. On exam questions, knowing which level is appropriate prevents you from under-treating items that need higher-level processing or overusing sterilization where it's not required.

Environmental cleaning includes wiping down exam tables, counters, and frequently touched surfaces between patients with appropriate disinfectants. It also involves managing the flow of "clean" and "dirty" items so that contaminated materials don't mix with sterile supplies. In a busy clinic, it can be tempting to shorten cleaning steps, but the exam expects you to prioritize proper disinfection even when you are behind. Correct answers typically involve following written protocols and giving disinfectants appropriate contact time.

4.5 Surgical Asepsis and Sterile Technique in the Office

SURGICAL ASEPSIS AIMS to keep an area completely free of microorganisms during invasive procedures. Even in outpatient settings, minor surgeries and invasive procedures require sterile technique. The CMA often helps set up and maintain this sterile field.

- Principles of maintaining a sterile field
- CMA responsibilities during minor surgical or sterile procedures

Maintaining a sterile field means that everything within the designated area must remain free from contamination. Sterile items can only touch other sterile items, and non-sterile items must be kept out of the field. Movement around the field should be controlled to avoid reaching over or turning your back on sterile areas. On the exam, breaking sterile technique—even accidentally—usually requires discarding contaminated items and starting over.

The CMA's responsibilities may include opening sterile packages correctly, adding sterile items to the field, and assisting the provider without contaminating equipment. You may also help prepare the patient's skin with appropriate antiseptics and position them for the procedure. During the procedure, you must be vigilant for any breaks in sterility and speak up if they occur. Exam scenarios where the CMA notices contamination but says nothing are testing whether you prioritize patient safety over convenience or hierarchy.

4.6 Sharps Safety and Exposure Control

SHARPS SUCH AS NEEDLES and lancets are essential tools but carry significant risk for injury and transmission of bloodborne pathogens. The CMA frequently handles sharps and must follow strict safety rules. The exam often includes clear right and wrong ways to manage sharps.

- Safe handling and disposal of sharps
- Steps to take after an accidental exposure

Safe sharps handling means never recapping used needles, never bending or breaking sharps by hand, and disposing of them immediately in approved sharps containers. These containers should be puncture-resistant, leakproof, and located as close as possible to the point of use. You should never overfill a sharps container; it must be closed and replaced when it reaches the fill line. On exam questions, any option involving recapping, carrying used sharps across the room, or placing them in regular trash should raise a red flag.

If an accidental exposure occurs—such as a needle-stick or splash of blood to mucous membranes—you must act quickly. Initial steps typically include washing the area with soap and water or flushing the eyes with clean water or saline, then reporting the incident immediately to a supervisor. An exposure report and follow-up evaluation, including possible baseline labs and post-exposure prophylaxis, may be required according to protocol. The exam favors answers that treat exposures as urgent events requiring prompt reporting and follow-up, not something to ignore.

4.7 Waste Management and Environmental Safety

PROPER DISPOSAL OF medical waste protects patients, staff, and the environment. The CMA needs to know what belongs in regular trash, biohazard containers, or sharps containers. Environmental safety also includes recognizing and addressing physical hazards in the clinic.

- Biohazard vs. regular waste classification
- Identifying and correcting environmental safety risks

Biohazard waste includes items contaminated with blood or certain body fluids, such as saturated gauze, used gloves from certain procedures, and specific cultures or specimens. These materials must be placed in designated biohazard bags or containers that are clearly labeled. Regular waste includes items like paper, wrappers, and some lightly contaminated materials that do not meet the threshold for biohazard classification, depending on facility policy. Exam questions will often test whether you can correctly sort items like used dressings, gloves, and sharps into the right containers.

Environmental safety risks include wet floors, loose cords, improperly stored equipment, or blocked exits that could lead to falls or injuries. As a CMA, you share responsibility for noticing and addressing these hazards promptly, such as cleaning spills, placing caution signs, or moving obstacles. You should also follow protocols for fire safety and emergency evacuation. On the exam, correct answers typically involve taking immediate steps to reduce risk and notifying appropriate staff rather than ignoring hazards.

4.8 Employee Health, Immunizations, and OSHA

PROTECTING EMPLOYEE health is a critical part of infection control. Immunizations, health screenings, and training all help reduce risk. OSHA (Occupational Safety and Health Administration) sets standards related to workplace safety and exposure to bloodborne pathogens that affect your daily practice.

- Role of employee immunizations and screenings
- OSHA-related responsibilities in the outpatient setting

Employee immunizations—such as those for hepatitis B, influenza, and other recommended vaccines—reduce the chance of staff acquiring or transmitting infections. Some facilities may require proof of immunity or offer vaccines as part of employment. Health screenings, such as TB testing, help identify potential risks early. On the exam, answers that support staff vaccination and appropriate screening align with best practices for infection control.

OSHA standards require employers to provide training, personal protective equipment, and an exposure control plan for workers at risk of contact with blood or other potentially infectious materials. As a CMA, you are expected to follow that plan, use PPE correctly, and participate in required training. You should also know how to access safety data sheets (SDS) and understand hazard labels. Questions that involve ignoring OSHA-related policies or refusing to use provided PPE are usually testing whether you recognize your responsibility to follow safety regulations.

4.9 Response to Spills, Accidents, and Exposure Incidents

SPILLS, ACCIDENTS, and exposure incidents are inevitable in healthcare settings, but they must be handled in a structured way. The CMA plays a key role in ensuring that responses are safe, prompt, and in line with policy. The exam will often present small "crisis" scenarios to see if you know the correct sequence of steps.

- Cleaning and containing blood or body fluid spills
- Reporting and documenting accidents and exposure incidents

Cleaning a blood or body fluid spill usually involves wearing appropriate PPE, containing the area, and using an approved disinfectant with sufficient contact time. You may need to block off the area to prevent others from walking through the spill. After cleaning, materials must be disposed of in appropriate waste containers. Exam questions typically favor answers that prioritize PPE, containment, and proper disinfectant use over quick, unprotected cleanup.

Accidents and exposures should be reported immediately according to facility policy. This may involve notifying a supervisor, completing incident or exposure forms, and arranging follow-up evaluation for those involved. Documentation should be factual and specific about what happened, without assigning blame or speculating. The exam tends to reward answers that treat these events as important safety issues, not minor inconveniences to hide or minimize.

4.10 Patient Education on Infection Prevention and Safety

PATIENTS ARE PARTNERS in infection prevention and safety. As a CMA, you often provide education on topics like handwashing, respiratory etiquette, wound care, and safe medication use. The exam tests whether you can explain these concepts clearly at a patient's level.

- Teaching hand hygiene, respiratory etiquette, and home care
- Explaining when to seek medical help or report concerns

Teaching hand hygiene may involve showing patients how to wash hands effectively, including scrubbing all surfaces and rinsing thoroughly. Respiratory etiquette includes covering coughs and sneezes, using tissues or the elbow, and safely disposing of used tissues. For home care, you may explain how to keep wounds clean, change dressings, or handle medications without contaminating them. On exam questions, effective teaching uses simple language, demonstrations, and checks for understanding.

Explaining when to seek medical help means giving clear instructions about warning signs that require prompt attention, such as increasing redness, swelling, fever, or drainage at a wound site. You might also advise patients to report side effects of medications or symptoms of infection that worsen rather than improve. Providing specific examples—like "call us if your fever is above X" or "go to the emergency room if you have trouble breathing"—helps patients know what to do. The exam favors answers where education is practical, concrete, and tailored to the patient's situation.

Practice Questions – Chapter 4 (25 Questions)

THESE QUESTIONS FOCUS on Chapter 4 topics: chain of infection, Standard and transmission-based precautions, asepsis, sterile technique, sharps safety, waste management, OSHA, spills/incidents, and patient education.

1. The "mode of transmission" in the chain of infection refers to:
   A. Where the microorganism lives and multiplies
   B. How the microorganism moves from one host to another
   C. How susceptible the host is to illness
   D. The specific symptoms caused
2. Hand hygiene primarily interrupts which link in the chain of infection?
   A. Infectious agent
   B. Reservoir
   C. Mode of transmission

D. Susceptible host

3. Standard Precautions apply to:
   A. Only patients with known infections
   B. Only hospitalized patients
   C. All patients, regardless of suspected infection status
   D. Only patients in isolation
4. In which situation is **soap and water** preferred over alcohol-based hand rub?
   A. Before entering the waiting room
   B. After removing clean gloves with no contamination
   C. When hands are visibly soiled
   D. Before using the computer
5. Which action best follows sharps safety guidelines?
   A. Recapping a used needle with two hands
   B. Throwing used sharps into a regular trash can
   C. Placing a used needle directly into a sharps container immediately after use
   D. Carrying the used needle across the room to dispose of later
6. A patient with suspected tuberculosis is scheduled for an exam. Which type of precautions is most appropriate?
   A. Contact
   B. Droplet
   C. Airborne
   D. Standard only
7. Which PPE is **most appropriate** for caring for a patient on contact precautions due to a draining wound?
   A. Gloves and gown
   B. Surgical mask only
   C. N95 respirator only
   D. No PPE is needed
8. An exam table is visibly soiled with blood after a procedure. The CMA should:
   A. Wipe it with a dry towel only
   B. Cover it with new paper and use it for the next patient
   C. Clean and disinfect the surface using an approved disinfectant and appropriate contact time
   D. Wait until the end of the day to clean it
9. Which statement best describes **medical asepsis**?
   A. Complete destruction of all microorganisms including spores
   B. Practices that reduce the number of microorganisms to safe levels
   C. Procedures used only in operating rooms
   D. The use of antibiotics for every patient
10. When assisting with a minor surgical procedure, the CMA notices the provider accidentally touches a non-sterile area with a sterile instrument. What is the **best** action?
   A. Ignore it to avoid delaying the procedure
   B. Quietly replace the instrument without telling anyone
   C. Inform the provider that sterility may have been broken and obtain a new sterile instrument
   D. Continue as usual and clean the instrument later
11. A sharps container is three-quarters full. The CMA should:

A. Continue using it until it is completely full
B. Overfill it to reduce the number of containers used
C. Close and replace the container according to policy
D. Shake it down to make more room

12. Biohazard waste includes:
A. Unsigned consent forms
B. Paper wrappers from sterile supplies
C. Gauze pads saturated with blood
D. Empty medication boxes

13. A CMA sustains a needle-stick injury after giving an injection. What is the **first** action they should take?
A. Tell no one and continue working
B. Wash the area with soap and water
C. Immediately leave work for the day
D. Post about it on social media

14. After an exposure incident such as a needle-stick, the CMA should:
A. Report the incident and complete required documentation
B. Ignore it if the patient seems healthy
C. Wait a week to see if they feel sick
D. Ask a coworker for advice instead of reporting

15. OSHA requires that facilities with bloodborne pathogen risk have:
A. No written policies to reduce paperwork
B. An exposure control plan and appropriate training for employees
C. Patient consent before using PPE
D. Only one sharps container per building

16. Which of the following actions demonstrates proper handling of a blood or body fluid spill?
A. Cleaning it with bare hands to work quickly
B. Placing a chair over it and leaving it
C. Wearing PPE, containing the area, and using approved disinfectant
D. Asking a patient to help clean it

17. A patient throws used tissues with visible nasal secretions into a regular trash can in the exam room. The CMA should:
A. Move the trash bag into a biohazard container if required by policy and encourage proper respiratory etiquette
B. Ignore the tissues
C. Put tissues back on the counter
D. Reuse the tissues to save supplies

18. Which statement about employee immunizations is most accurate?
A. They are irrelevant to infection control
B. They help protect both staff and patients from certain infections
C. They are only for pediatric staff
D. They replace the need for Standard Precautions

19. A patient asks how to prevent infection in a new surgical wound at home. The most appropriate CMA response is to:
A. Tell them not to touch the wound at all

B. Give clear instructions on handwashing, dressing changes, and signs of infection to watch for
C. Suggest they use any home remedy they prefer
D. Say "just keep it clean" without details

20. A patient with diarrhea is placed in an exam room. To reduce environmental contamination, the CMA should:
A. Leave the door open so air circulates
B. Ensure surfaces are disinfected after the visit and handle waste according to policy
C. Use only dry wipes on surfaces
D. Avoid cleaning to prevent aerosolization
21. Which behavior best demonstrates **respiratory etiquette**?
A. Coughing into one's hand and touching surfaces
B. Sneezing into the air away from others
C. Coughing into the elbow or a tissue and disposing of the tissue properly
D. Removing masks to cough more comfortably
22. A CMA notes an extension cord stretched across a hallway where patients walk. What should they do?
A. Step over it carefully and move on
B. Move the cord or mark the area and notify appropriate staff to correct the hazard
C. Tell patients to watch their step without changing anything
D. Unplug all equipment without telling anyone
23. A patient is placed on droplet precautions. Which of the following is most appropriate when entering the room?
A. Wearing gloves only
B. Wearing a surgical mask within the recommended distance of the patient
C. Wearing an N95 respirator only
D. Wearing no PPE
24. A patient asks, "When should I call the clinic after I go home?" Which response best supports safety?
A. "Only call if you have pain."
B. "Call if you have increasing redness, swelling, fever, or drainage, or if you're worried something isn't right."
C. "Don't call; just go to the emergency room for everything."
D. "You shouldn't need to call us."
25. A CMA is tempted to skip disinfecting an exam table between patients because the schedule is behind. From an exam perspective, this option is:
A. Acceptable if the patient looks healthy
B. Acceptable if the next patient doesn't mind
C. Unsafe and inconsistent with infection-control standards
D. Required to keep the schedule on time

Answer Key – Chapter 4 (with Justifications)

1. **B** – Mode of transmission describes how the microorganism moves from one host to another (e.g., contact, droplet, airborne).
2. **C** – Hand hygiene primarily interrupts the mode of transmission by removing organisms before they can move to another host.
3. **C** – Standard Precautions are applied to all patients regardless of known or suspected infection status.

4. **C** – Soap and water are preferred when hands are visibly soiled or contaminated with certain organisms.
5. **C** – Used sharps should be placed directly into an approved sharps container immediately after use; recapping or using regular trash is unsafe.
6. **C** – Suspected tuberculosis requires airborne precautions due to airborne transmission of the organism.
7. **A** – Gloves and gown are appropriate for contact precautions when dealing with draining wounds to prevent spread via direct contact.
8. **C** – Visible blood requires cleaning and disinfection with an approved product and proper contact time before the next patient uses the table.
9. **B** – Medical asepsis involves practices that reduce microorganisms to safe levels, not complete sterilization.
10. **C** – Breaking sterile technique requires addressing the contamination; informing the provider and obtaining a new sterile instrument protects patient safety.
11. **C** – Sharps containers should be closed and replaced when near the fill line (often around three-quarters full) to prevent overfilling and injury.
12. **C** – Gauze pads saturated with blood are considered biohazard waste and must be placed in appropriate containers.
13. **B** – The first step after a needle-stick is to wash the area with soap and water to reduce contamination, followed by reporting.
14. **A** – Exposure incidents must be reported and documented according to policy to ensure proper evaluation and follow-up.
15. **B** – OSHA requires an exposure control plan, training, and appropriate protective measures in workplaces with bloodborne pathogen risks.
16. **C** – Wearing PPE, containing the area, and using approved disinfectant with proper contact time is the correct way to manage spills.
17. **A** – Depending on policy, tissues with visible secretions may be managed as potentially infectious; the CMA should also reinforce proper respiratory etiquette.
18. **B** – Employee immunizations help protect both staff and patients from certain infections, forming part of infection control.
19. **B** – Providing specific instructions on hygiene, dressing changes, and warning signs helps patients prevent infection and know when to seek help.
20. **B** – Disinfecting surfaces and handling waste properly helps reduce environmental contamination in cases like diarrhea.
21. **C** – Coughing into the elbow or a tissue and disposing of the tissue properly is good respiratory etiquette and reduces spread.
22. **B** – Addressing the tripping hazard by moving or marking the cord and notifying appropriate staff reduces risk of falls.
23. **B** – Droplet precautions require a surgical mask when within the recommended distance of the patient to block large respiratory droplets.
24. **B** – Giving specific signs like redness, swelling, fever, or drainage and inviting the patient to call if worried supports safety and clarity.
25. **C** – Skipping disinfection between patients is unsafe and violates infection-control standards, regardless of schedule pressure.

Chapter 5

Patient Assessment and Vital Signs

Patient assessment is often the first step in every visit, and vital signs provide quick, objective information about how a patient is doing. As a CMA, you're frequently the person gathering this data and communicating it to the provider. This chapter focuses on how to collect accurate information, measure and interpret vital signs, and recognize when something is urgent.

5.1 The Role of the CMA in Patient Assessment

THE CMA PLAYS A CENTRAL role in the initial assessment of patients during office visits. You are often the first clinical staff member to interact with the patient, so the information you collect sets the tone for the entire encounter. The exam tests whether you understand what falls within your assessment responsibilities and how to handle that information.

- Gathering preliminary data and chief complaint
- Recognizing abnormal findings and reporting appropriately

Gathering preliminary data includes confirming patient identity, measuring vital signs, and documenting the chief complaint in the patient's own words. You may also review medication lists, allergies, and recent changes in health status. It's important to listen carefully and avoid inserting your own interpretation into the patient's description. On exam questions, correct answers show the CMA collecting accurate, objective data and recording it clearly in the chart.

Recognizing abnormal findings means you can identify when vital signs or symptoms fall outside expected ranges. You are not diagnosing, but you should know when something requires prompt attention from the provider or nurse. For example, very high blood pressure, difficulty breathing, or chest pain are red flags that must be reported immediately. The exam will often present you with abnormal findings and test whether you know to escalate rather than simply proceed with routine steps.

5.2 Subjective vs. Objective Data

ASSESSMENT DATA CAN be grouped into subjective information from the patient and objective findings you can measure or observe. Understanding the difference helps you document accurately and think like a member of the care team. The exam expects you to recognize which type of data you are dealing with in a given scenario.

- Subjective data: what the patient reports
- Objective data: what you can measure or observe

Subjective data includes the patient's description of pain, symptoms, feelings, or concerns—things that only they can truly know. For example, "I feel dizzy," "My pain is a 7 out of 10," or "I've been really tired" are subjective statements. You should document them as quotes or paraphrases that clearly reflect the patient's perspective. On the exam, trying to "correct" a patient's subjective report is usually a mistake; your role is to record it, not argue with it.

Objective data includes measurable or observable facts such as blood pressure, temperature, weight, respiratory rate, skin color, or visible swelling. These findings are the same regardless of who observes them, assuming proper technique.

When documenting objective data, you should avoid inserting your opinions and instead use descriptive language—e.g., “red, warm area on left calf” instead of “leg looks bad.” Exam questions often involve distinguishing whether a statement is subjective or objective and how it should be recorded.

5.3 Measuring Temperature Accurately

TEMPERATURE IS A KEY vital sign that helps identify infection, inflammation, and other conditions. Different routes—oral, tympanic, temporal, axillary, and rectal—have different techniques and typical values. The exam tests whether you know how to measure temperature accurately and interpret common variations.

- Common temperature routes and considerations
- Interpreting temperature readings and recognizing fever

Oral temperatures are common for cooperative adults and older children, but they can be affected by recent eating, drinking, or smoking. Tympanic (ear) and temporal (forehead) thermometers provide quicker readings but require correct placement to be accurate. Axillary temperatures (under the arm) are less invasive but tend to run slightly lower and may be less precise. Rectal temperatures are generally closest to core temperature but are invasive and used selectively; they are typically higher than oral readings. On exam questions, choosing the correct route often depends on the patient’s age, condition, and cooperation.

Interpreting temperature involves knowing the general normal range and what qualifies as fever. While exact “normal” can vary slightly, a reading significantly above baseline suggests possible infection or other problems. You should also consider other signs, such as chills, sweating, or flushed skin. When the exam presents a temperature and asks what to do, the safest answers often involve reporting concerning fevers to the provider and double-checking unusually low or high readings before acting on them.

5.4 Measuring Pulse and Recognizing Abnormalities

PULSE MEASUREMENT PROVIDES information about heart rate and rhythm. The CMA commonly checks radial pulses, but other sites like apical pulses may be used in certain situations. The exam will expect you to know how to measure pulse properly and recognize when it is abnormal.

- Pulse rate, rhythm, and quality
- Factors that can affect pulse readings

Pulse rate is the number of beats per minute, while rhythm refers to how regular or irregular the pattern is. Quality (or amplitude) describes how strong or weak the pulse feels. To measure a radial pulse, you place your first two or three fingers over the radial artery at the wrist and count beats for 30 seconds (and multiply by two) or 60 seconds for irregular rhythms. On exam questions, a pulse that is too fast, too slow, or irregular often requires you to notify the provider.

Factors that can affect pulse include exercise, stress, fever, medications, and underlying heart conditions. For example, beta blockers may slow the heart rate, while pain or anxiety may raise it. You should be aware of these influences when interpreting readings and documenting them. The exam often presents vital signs in context—for example, a high pulse in a patient with fever—and tests whether you recognize when the finding fits the situation or is concerning enough to report.

5.5 Measuring Respirations and Recognizing Distress

RESPIRATORY RATE AND pattern give important clues about a patient's breathing status. Because people may change their breathing if they know it's being measured, you often assess respirations discreetly. The exam uses respiratory questions to see whether you can spot signs of distress.

- Measuring respiratory rate and pattern
- Signs of respiratory distress that must be reported

To measure respiratory rate, you count the number of breaths per minute, usually while pretending to continue checking the pulse so the patient doesn't consciously alter their breathing. You also note whether breaths are regular, shallow, deep, or labored. Normal ranges vary with age, but you should have a general sense of what is expected for adults and children. On exam questions, respiratory rates that are markedly high or low usually signal a need for prompt provider notification.

Signs of respiratory distress include shortness of breath, use of accessory muscles (like neck muscles), nasal flaring, cyanosis (bluish lips or fingers), and difficulty speaking in full sentences. Patients in distress may sit upright, lean forward, or appear anxious. These signs indicate that breathing is compromised and require immediate attention, not routine processing. The exam often presents subtle clues—like a patient who can't finish sentences without pausing to breathe—and expects you to respond appropriately.

5.6 Blood Pressure Measurement and Errors

BLOOD PRESSURE REFLECTS the force of blood against artery walls and is crucial for identifying hypertension, hypotension, and other cardiovascular issues. Accurate measurement depends on correct cuff size, positioning, and technique. The exam frequently covers both procedure and interpretation.

- Proper technique for measuring blood pressure
- Common errors that can lead to inaccurate readings

Proper technique includes using the correct cuff size (bladder covering about 80% of the arm circumference), positioning the arm at heart level, and ensuring the patient is seated and rested. You place the cuff snugly on the bare upper arm, locate the brachial artery, and position the stethoscope over it. Inflate the cuff appropriately, then deflate at a steady rate while listening for Korotkoff sounds to determine systolic and diastolic pressures. Exam questions often describe parts of this process and ask which step was done incorrectly.

Common errors include using a cuff that is too small or too large, taking readings over clothing, or measuring while the patient is talking, moving, or has just exercised. These mistakes can falsely elevate or lower readings. Releasing air too quickly or not allowing the patient to rest before measurement can also skew results. On the exam, when you see an obviously wrong technique, the correct answer usually involves re-measuring with proper conditions rather than accepting a questionable reading.

5.7 Height, Weight, BMI, and Anthropometric Measurements

HEIGHT AND WEIGHT ARE basic measurements that support medication dosing, growth assessment, and evaluation of nutritional status. Body mass index (BMI) is a calculated value that estimates body fat based on height and weight. The exam may test your procedure for measuring these as well as your understanding of why they matter.

- Measuring height and weight accurately
- Basic understanding of BMI and growth considerations

Measuring height and weight requires using calibrated equipment and consistent procedures. Patients should remove heavy outer clothing and shoes for more accurate weight, and you should ensure they stand straight against the stadiometer for height. For infants and small children, length and weight may be measured lying down or using specialized pediatric scales. Exam questions may ask which step is needed to improve accuracy or which measurement method is correct for a given age group.

BMI is calculated using height and weight and categorized into ranges such as underweight, normal, overweight, and obese. While you are not responsible for diagnosing or counseling based solely on BMI, you may collect the data and enter it into the EHR for provider review. Growth charts are used for children to track development against age-based norms. On the exam, you might be asked to recognize when a measurement appears out of pattern—for example, a sudden jump or drop in pediatric growth curves—and to report it rather than interpret it.

5.8 Pain Assessment and Use of Pain Scales

PAIN IS OFTEN CALLED the "fifth vital sign" because of its importance in assessment. Unlike blood pressure or temperature, pain is inherently subjective and must be reported by the patient. The exam tests whether you can assess pain systematically and document it accurately.

- Using pain scales and patient self-report
- Documenting pain location, quality, and impact

Pain scales provide a structured way to quantify pain, such as 0–10 numeric scales for adults or visual faces scales for children or nonverbal patients. You ask the patient to rate their pain, emphasizing that there are no "right" or "wrong" answers. Reassessing pain after interventions is also important. Exam questions often include a patient rating ("8 out of 10") and expect you to document it and report significant pain to the provider rather than ignoring it.

Documenting pain should include location ("left lower back"), quality (sharp, dull, burning), duration, and any factors that worsen or relieve it. You may also note how pain affects daily activities, such as walking or sleeping. Objective observations—such as guarding, grimacing, or reluctance to move—can be recorded along with the patient's report. The exam rewards answers that combine subjective and objective data and treat the patient's self-report as valid information.

5.9 Special Considerations: Pediatrics, Geriatrics, and Pregnancy

DIFFERENT PATIENT POPULATIONS have specific assessment needs and vital sign norms. Pediatrics, older adults, and pregnant patients require special attention to technique, interpretation, and safety. The exam often draws from these groups to test whether you can adapt your approach.

- Pediatric assessment and age-based vital sign differences
- Geriatric and pregnancy-specific assessment considerations

In pediatric patients, vital sign ranges differ from adults; for example, infants typically have higher heart and respiratory rates. Measuring temperature may require different routes depending on age and cooperation. Weight and growth are monitored closely, often plotted on growth charts. Exam questions may ask which vital sign is most concerning for a particular age or which technique is most appropriate for a young child.

Geriatric patients may have changes in blood pressure regulation, temperature regulation, and pain expression. They might not present "classic" symptoms—for instance, an older adult with infection may have confusion rather than fever. Pregnant patients have physiological changes such as increased heart rate and altered blood pressure patterns. The exam may show you vital signs that are normal variations in pregnancy versus those that suggest complications, and it expects you to report concerning findings without making diagnoses.

5.10 Documentation, Trends, and When to Escalate

COLLECTING VITAL SIGNS and assessment data is only useful if it is documented accurately and used to detect trends. The CMA must chart findings clearly and recognize when changes over time indicate a problem. The exam often tests whether you act appropriately once you notice an abnormal pattern.

- Accurate documentation of vital signs and assessment data
- Recognizing trends and knowing when to notify the provider

Accurate documentation means recording each vital sign with units, time, and any relevant conditions—such as "BP 142/88 mmHg, sitting, left arm." You should avoid rounding excessively or estimating values, and you must correct mistakes according to policy rather than hiding them. Notes about patient behavior or symptoms should be objective and specific. On exam questions, the best answers usually involve clear, complete documentation that another clinician could understand without guessing.

Recognizing trends means comparing current readings to previous ones and looking for meaningful changes. A single slightly elevated blood pressure might be less concerning than a pattern of increasing readings over several visits. Sudden changes—like a rapid drop in blood pressure or spike in heart rate—can signal acute problems that need urgent attention. The exam expects you to notify the provider when trends or values suggest risk, rather than just filing the numbers away.

Practice Questions – Chapter 5 (25 Questions)

THESE QUESTIONS FOCUS on Chapter 5 topics: CMA role in assessment, subjective vs objective data, temperature, pulse, respirations, blood pressure, anthropometrics, pain, special populations, documentation, and escalation.

1. A patient states, "My chest feels tight, and I'm short of breath." This information is best described as:
   A. Objective data
   B. Subjective data
   C. Diagnostic data
   D. Irrelevant data

2. Which of the following is **objective** data?
   A. "I feel really tired lately."
   B. "My pain is a 9 out of 10."
   C. BP 150/94 mmHg, sitting, right arm
   D. "I'm worried about my results."
3. When documenting the chief complaint, the CMA should:
   A. Interpret the complaint in medical terms without quoting the patient
   B. Record it using the patient's own words as much as possible
   C. Only document the provider's interpretation
   D. Skip it if the visit reason is obvious
4. A patient drank hot coffee 5 minutes ago. The CMA needs to take an oral temperature. What is the **best** action?
   A. Take the temperature immediately
   B. Wait 15–20 minutes before taking the oral temperature
   C. Ask the patient to drink cold water, then take the temperature
   D. Switch to oral temperature on the other side of the mouth
5. Which temperature route is generally closest to core body temperature and typically slightly higher than oral readings?
   A. Temporal
   B. Axillary
   C. Rectal
   D. Tympanic
6. When measuring a radial pulse, the CMA should:
   A. Use their thumb to feel the pulse
   B. Count the beats for 15 seconds and multiply by four for all patients
   C. Use the first two or three fingers and count for a full minute if the rhythm is irregular
   D. Press so hard that the pulse disappears
7. A patient's pulse is 120 beats per minute at rest. The CMA's **most appropriate** action is to:
   A. Ignore it and continue with the visit
   B. Document the finding and promptly notify the provider
   C. Record it as normal
   D. Tell the patient to go home and rest
8. Which technique is best for measuring respiratory rate?
   A. Watching the chest rise and fall after telling the patient you are counting breaths
   B. Counting respirations while pretending to continue checking the pulse
   C. Asking the patient to count their own breaths
   D. Estimating based on how fast they are talking
9. A patient is breathing rapidly, using neck muscles, and can only speak in short phrases. This suggests:
   A. Mild anxiety, no concern
   B. Normal variation
   C. Respiratory distress that requires prompt provider notification
   D. Sleepiness
10. When measuring blood pressure, the cuff should:
    A. Be placed over clothing for comfort

B. Be too loose so it can slide
C. Fit so the bladder covers about 80% of the arm circumference
D. Be inflated until the patient feels pain

11. Which error is most likely to cause a falsely **high** blood pressure reading?
A. Using a cuff that is too large
B. Using a cuff that is too small
C. Allowing the patient to rest quietly before measurement
D. Positioning the arm at heart level

12. Before taking blood pressure, the CMA should **first**:
A. Have the patient walk briskly to get an accurate reading
B. Ensure the patient is seated, relaxed, and has rested a few minutes
C. Ask the patient to talk continuously
D. Take the reading while the patient is standing and moving

13. When measuring weight, the CMA should:
A. Ask the patient to keep shoes and heavy outerwear on
B. Use a calibrated scale and have the patient remove heavy clothing and shoes if possible
C. Estimate the weight if the patient is in a hurry
D. Only weigh patients who request it

14. A child's weight suddenly drops from the 50th percentile to the 10th percentile on the growth chart over a short period. The CMA should:
A. Ignore it; growth charts are not important
B. Document the change and bring it to the provider's attention
C. Diagnose malnutrition
D. Alter the chart to keep the percentile stable

15. An adult patient reports "severe pain" and rates it as 9/10. The CMA's **best** response is to:
A. Tell them it can't be that bad
B. Document the pain scale, location, and characteristics and notify the provider
C. Reduce the number to 5/10 in the chart
D. Ignore the pain because the patient looks comfortable

16. When using a faces pain scale for a young child, the CMA should:
A. Tell the child which face to choose
B. Ask the child to point to the face that shows how they feel
C. Use it only if the child can read numbers
D. Avoid asking about pain

17. Which of the following findings in an older adult is **most concerning** and requires prompt reporting?
A. Slightly lower temperature than expected
B. Mild stiffness upon waking
C. New confusion and disorientation compared with baseline
D. Preference for sitting instead of standing

18. A pregnant patient at a routine visit has a slightly higher heart rate than her pre-pregnancy baseline but feels well. The CMA should:
A. Recognize this can be a normal change in pregnancy and document it
B. Assume she is having a heart attack
C. Refuse to take any more vital signs

D. Ignore the heart rate completely

19. A patient's blood pressure has increased from 128/78 mmHg at several previous visits to 160/100 mmHg today. The CMA should:
    A. Document and notify the provider promptly because of the significant rise
    B. Change today's reading to match previous values
    C. Assume the patient is just anxious and ignore it
    D. Tell the patient there is no reason for concern
20. Which documentation entry is most appropriate for vital signs?
    A. "Vitals normal."
    B. "BP fine, pulse ok."
    C. "BP 138/86 mmHg, sitting, left arm; P 92 bpm, regular; R 18/min, unlabored; T 98.7°F oral."
    D. "Everything looks good."
21. A patient with a history of hypertension refuses to have their blood pressure taken. What should the CMA do?
    A. Force the patient to comply
    B. Respect the refusal, document it, and notify the provider
    C. Fake a reading in the chart
    D. Cancel the visit without telling anyone
22. A pediatric patient is crying loudly during vital signs. The CMA should:
    A. Recognize that crying can affect some vital signs and note this when reporting
    B. Ignore the crying and assume readings are perfect
    C. Yell at the child to be quiet
    D. Skip vital signs entirely
23. A CMA repeats a blood pressure that seemed unusually low and gets a similar result. The **next** best step is to:
    A. Discard both readings and stop measuring
    B. Document the values clearly and notify the provider
    C. Change the values to a normal number
    D. Ask the patient to stand up quickly and see if they feel dizzy
24. A patient reports dizziness when standing up quickly. Which vital sign measurement is most directly helpful to assess this complaint?
    A. Oral temperature
    B. Orthostatic blood pressures and pulses (lying and standing)
    C. Weight
    D. BMI
25. A CMA notices that a patient's respiratory rate has gradually increased over the last three visits, and today the patient also reports new shortness of breath. The **best** action is to:
    A. Ignore the trend since each rate is within general normal limits
    B. Document and highlight the trend and symptoms, then notify the provider
    C. Only document today's rate and ignore prior ones
    D. Tell the patient to monitor breathing at home without informing anyone

Answer Key – Chapter 5 (with Justifications)

1. **B** – The patient's description of chest tightness and shortness of breath is subjective data because it comes

from their personal experience.

2. **C** – Blood pressure with specific numbers and conditions is objective data, as it is measurable and observable by others.
3. **B** – Chief complaints should be recorded using the patient's own words as much as possible to accurately reflect their concerns.
4. **B** – Hot or cold drinks can affect oral temperature readings; waiting 15–20 minutes helps ensure accuracy.
5. **C** – Rectal temperatures are typically closest to core temperature and usually slightly higher than oral readings.
6. **C** – The first two or three fingers (not the thumb) are used for pulse, and a full minute count is best when the rhythm is irregular.
7. **B** – A resting pulse of 120 bpm is elevated and should be documented and reported promptly to the provider for evaluation.
8. **B** – Counting respirations discreetly while pretending to check the pulse helps avoid altering the patient's natural breathing pattern.
9. **C** – Rapid breathing, use of accessory muscles, and difficulty speaking suggest respiratory distress needing prompt attention.
10. **C** – The cuff bladder should cover about 80% of the arm circumference to obtain an accurate blood pressure reading.
11. **B** – A cuff that is too small can cause falsely high readings because it exerts more pressure on a smaller area.
12. **B** – The patient should be seated, relaxed, and rested a few minutes before taking blood pressure to improve accuracy.
13. **B** – Accurate weights require a calibrated scale and removal of heavy clothing and shoes whenever possible.
14. **B** – A significant drop in growth percentile should be documented and brought to the provider's attention for further evaluation.
15. **B** – The CMA should respect the patient's report, document pain details, and notify the provider rather than minimizing or altering the rating.
16. **B** – Faces scales are designed for children; asking them to point to the face that matches how they feel is appropriate.
17. **C** – New confusion or disorientation in an older adult is concerning and may signal serious conditions like infection or stroke.
18. **A** – Slightly increased heart rate can be a normal physiologic change in pregnancy; the CMA should document it and report anything worrisome.
19. **A** – A jump from 128/78 to 160/100 is significant and should be documented and reported promptly to the provider.
20. **C** – This entry includes full vital sign values, units, positions, and conditions, which supports clear communication and trend analysis.
21. **B** – Patients have the right to refuse; the CMA should document the refusal and inform the provider rather than falsifying data.
22. **A** – Crying can affect heart rate, respirations, and sometimes blood pressure; noting this context when reporting is important.
23. **B** – Repeated low readings that are consistent should be documented and promptly reported to the provider, not altered or ignored.
24. **B** – Orthostatic blood pressures and pulses (lying and standing) help assess dizziness related to position changes.

25. **B** – A rising respiratory rate trend plus new shortness of breath suggests potential deterioration and should be documented and reported.

Chapter 6

Pharmacology, Medications, and Immunizations

Medications and vaccines are a huge part of outpatient practice, and CMAs are often deeply involved in handling, preparing, and administering them under provider orders. The CMA exam expects you to know basic pharmacology concepts, safe medication practices, and core immunization principles. This chapter focuses on what you must know to keep patients safe while staying firmly within your scope of practice.

6.1 The CMA's Role in Medication Management

CMAS SUPPORT MEDICATION management but do **not** prescribe or independently change therapies. You work under the direction of licensed providers and follow protocols carefully. The exam frequently tests whether you recognize your role and stay within your boundaries.

- Permitted tasks under delegation
- Tasks that remain outside CMA scope

Permitted tasks typically include verifying patient identity, preparing medications as ordered, administering certain medications (where allowed by law and facility policy), and documenting what was given. You may also collect information about current medications, allergies, and over-the-counter or herbal products. In some settings, you might be allowed to call in prescriptions that the provider has authorized or send e-prescriptions for signature. Exam questions reward answers that show you following explicit orders and policies rather than improvising.

Tasks outside CMA scope include prescribing medications, changing dosages on your own, or deciding to start or stop a medication without provider input. You also may not diagnose conditions or guarantee outcomes of treatments. When in doubt, the safest exam answer usually involves checking with the provider or licensed nurse. The test often includes tempting options—like "just adjust the insulin dose for the patient"—that are incorrect because they cross into provider-level decisions.

6.2 Basic Pharmacology: Drug Names and Classifications

PHARMACOLOGY BASICS help you understand what medications do and how they are organized. While CMAs are not expected to be pharmacists, you should recognize common naming conventions and major drug categories. The exam uses these basics to see if you can safely handle and talk about medications.

- Generic vs. brand names
- Drug classes and therapeutic categories

Generic names are the official, nonproprietary names of medications, while brand (or trade) names are created by manufacturers and often capitalized. For example, one drug may have many brand names but only one generic name. In practice, providers and pharmacies may use either, so you should recognize both formats. Exam questions may ask which name type is which or which name is standardized versus tied to a specific company.

Drug classes group medications by how they work or what they treat—like antihypertensives, antibiotics, or bronchodilators. Knowing the class can give you clues about expected effects and common side effects, even if you haven't seen a specific drug before. For example, many beta blockers share similar names and actions. On the exam, recognizing the class may help you answer questions about why a drug is ordered or what to monitor, without requiring detailed memorization of every product.

6.3 Pharmacokinetics and Pharmacodynamics (High-Level)

PHARMACOKINETICS DESCRIBES what the body does to a drug, and pharmacodynamics describes what the drug does to the body. The CMA exam only expects a high-level understanding, but these ideas can explain why dosing and timing matter. Thinking this way helps you appreciate why safety steps exist.

- Absorption, distribution, metabolism, and excretion (ADME)
- Drug actions: therapeutic effects and side effects

Absorption is how a drug enters the bloodstream—for example, through the GI tract, skin, muscle, or directly into a vein. Distribution describes how it travels around the body, metabolism, how it is broken down (often in the liver), and excretion of how it leaves (often through the kidneys). These processes affect how quickly a medication works, how long it lasts, and how often it must be given. Exam questions may ask general questions like why renal or liver disease might affect medication handling.

Drug actions include the desired therapeutic effects (such as lowering blood pressure or reducing pain) and possible side effects or adverse reactions. Therapeutic effects are why the drug is prescribed, while side effects are additional, sometimes unwanted, effects that may be mild or serious. You must be alert for patient reports of unusual symptoms after starting or changing a medication. On the exam, safe answers usually involve recognizing concerning side effects and notifying the provider rather than dismissing them.

6.4 Medication Orders, Labels, and the "Rights" of Medication Administration

SAFE MEDICATION PRACTICE starts with a clear order and correct interpretation of labels. The CMA must understand each part of a medication order and follow the "rights" of administration. The exam uses these concepts heavily in safety-focused questions.

- Components of a complete medication order and label
- The medication "rights" as safety checks

A complete medication order typically includes the patient's name, medication name, dosage, route, frequency, and provider's signature (plus date/time). Labels on medication containers list the drug name, strength, dosage form, expiration date, and storage instructions. Reading labels carefully helps prevent errors—confusing similar-looking names or strengths can be dangerous. On exam questions, incomplete or unclear orders should be clarified with the provider before administration.

The "rights" of medication administration—commonly the right patient, right drug, right dose, right route, right time, and right documentation—act as a mental checklist. Some organizations add more rights, like right reason, right response, or right education. For the CMA, consistently applying these rights means verifying identity, checking labels against orders, and documenting immediately after administration. Exam answers that skip or rush through these checks often represent unsafe practice.

6.5 Routes of Administration and Forms of Medications

MEDICATIONS CAN BE given by many routes, and forms like tablets, liquids, or injections are chosen based on patient needs and drug properties. The CMA exam expects you to understand common routes and how they affect practice. Technique and safety vary with each route.

- Common routes: oral, topical, inhalation, and parenteral
- Forms of medications (tablets, capsules, solutions, suspensions, etc.)

Oral medications are taken by mouth and swallowed, often in tablet or capsule form, and are convenient for many patients. Topical medications are applied to the skin or mucous membranes as creams, ointments, or patches. Inhalation medications deliver drugs directly to the respiratory tract via inhalers or nebulizers. Parenteral routes (such as intramuscular, subcutaneous, or intradermal) involve injections and generally act more quickly. Exam questions may ask which route is most appropriate in a scenario or what precautions are needed for each.

Medication forms include tablets (solid, often swallowable), capsules (shells containing powder or liquid), solutions (clear liquids with dissolved drug), suspensions (liquids with particles that must be shaken), and others like patches or suppositories. Some tablets are extended-release or enteric-coated and must not be crushed or split. On the exam, correct answers often involve recognizing instructions like "do not crush" or understanding that suspensions must be shaken before dosing to avoid unequal medication distribution.

6.6 Safe Medication Administration and Calculation Awareness

WHILE CMAS MAY NOT perform complex calculations in all settings, you must be aware of basic dosing concepts and recognize when something seems unsafe. The exam may test basic math awareness conceptually, but it strongly emphasizes safe behavior. When in doubt, double-check and ask.

- Double-checking doses, units, and calculations
- Recognizing potential dosing errors and near misses

Double-checking doses means comparing the order to the label and ensuring the units match (mg vs. mcg, mL vs. tsp, etc.). Even simple errors—like misreading a decimal point—can have serious consequences. In many clinics, high-risk medications require a second check by another staff member or the provider. On exam questions, rushing through calculations or ignoring unit mismatches is a red flag; safer answers involve slowing down and verifying.

Recognizing potential dosing errors includes being suspicious of unusually large or small doses, incorrect routes, or orders that don't fit the patient's age or condition. For example, an adult dose ordered for a small child may be inappropriate. Near misses—errors caught before reaching the patient—should still be reported according to policy so systems can improve. The test often favors answers where the CMA questions an order politely and seeks clarification instead of administering a dose they don't understand.

6.7 High-Alert Medications and Allergy Considerations

SOME MEDICATIONS CARRY higher risks and are considered "high-alert" because errors with them can cause serious harm. Allergies are another critical safety concern that must be checked before any drug is given. The CMA exam expects you to treat both issues with extra caution.

- Recognizing high-alert medications conceptually
- Verifying and documenting allergies and reactions

High-alert medications include things like insulin, certain anticoagulants, some cardiac drugs, and others identified by facility lists and safety organizations. You may not need to memorize every drug, but you should know that these require extra checks and careful monitoring. In exam questions, a scenario involving a high-risk medication often tests whether you follow protocols precisely and confirm orders instead of taking shortcuts.

Allergy verification is essential at every visit, especially before medication administration. You should ask about medication allergies and what kind of reaction occurred ("rash," "trouble breathing," etc.), then document clearly. It's also important to distinguish between side effects and true allergies; for example, mild stomach upset may not be a true allergy. However, on the exam, you treat reported allergies seriously and never give a medication that the patient is listed as allergic to without explicit provider review and clarification.

6.8 Immunization Basics: Principles and Schedules

IMMUNIZATIONS ARE A core part of preventive care in outpatient settings. CMAs often help with vaccine screening, preparation, and administration under provider orders. The exam expects a general understanding of vaccine principles and safe practices, not memorization of every schedule detail.

- Purpose and basic concept of immunizations
- General awareness of routine vaccine schedules and documentation

Immunizations work by stimulating the immune system to recognize and respond to specific pathogens without causing the full-blown disease. They can significantly reduce the risk of infection and community spread. Some vaccines require multiple doses over time to achieve full protection, and boosters may be needed. On exam questions, you may be asked why vaccinations are important or to choose correct patient education points.

Routine vaccine schedules differ by age group—infants and children receive a series of vaccines at well-child visits, while adults may need boosters (such as tetanus) and specific vaccines based on risk (like influenza or pneumonia). CMAs assist by checking records, ensuring the right vaccine is given at the right age and interval, and documenting the lot number, manufacturer, and site of administration. The exam often includes questions on what should be recorded for a vaccine and the importance of maintaining accurate immunization histories.

6.9 Vaccine Screening, Storage, and Administration Safety

VACCINES MUST BE STORED, handled, and administered correctly to remain effective and safe. Screening helps identify contraindications or precautions before giving a vaccine. The exam tests whether you understand these safety steps and follow them carefully.

- Screening for contraindications and precautions
- Proper storage, handling, and administration practices

Screening questions may include asking about previous severe reactions to vaccines, current illness, allergies (especially to components like eggs or gelatin, depending on the vaccine), and specific conditions such as pregnancy or immunosuppression. If screening suggests a potential contraindication, the provider must review the situation before proceeding. In exam scenarios, administering a vaccine despite red-flag screening responses is usually the wrong choice; the safe answer involves pausing and consulting the provider.

Proper storage typically requires maintaining vaccines within certain temperature ranges in monitored refrigerators or freezers, and never storing them in areas like regular food fridges that lack proper controls. Handling includes protecting vaccines from light if needed, rotating stock by expiration date, and preparing doses immediately before use. Administration safety involves using correct routes (IM, SubQ, etc.), sites (like deltoid or anterolateral thigh by age), and needle sizes according to guidelines and policy. Exam questions often test your understanding of route/site matching and the importance of not using expired or improperly stored vaccines.

6.10 Patient Education and Medication/Vaccine Teaching

PATIENT EDUCATION IS a key CMA responsibility related to medications and immunizations. You help patients understand how and when to take medications and what to expect after vaccines. The exam frequently includes teaching scenarios to see whether your explanations are safe and clear.

- Teaching about medication use, adherence, and side effects
- Teaching about expected vaccine reactions and when to seek help

Medication teaching includes explaining how to take medications (with or without food if specified), the importance of following the schedule, and what to do if doses are missed—usually referring to provider or pharmacy guidance. You should instruct patients not to change doses or stop medications without talking to the provider. Discussing common, non-dangerous side effects in simple terms and warning signs that require medical attention helps patients manage therapy safely. Exam answers that encourage adherence and refer complex questions back to the provider are usually correct.

Vaccine teaching should cover minor expected reactions—such as soreness at the injection site, mild fever, or fatigue—and simple comfort measures like cool compresses if permitted by policy. You should also discuss serious warning signs, such as difficulty breathing, swelling of face or throat, or high fever, and instruct patients or parents to seek immediate care if these occur. Clear guidance about when to call the clinic versus when to go to emergency care improves safety. The exam favors patient education that is specific, realistic, and avoids minimizing concerns.

Practice Questions – Chapter 6 (25 Questions)

THESE QUESTIONS FOCUS on Chapter 6 topics: CMA role/scope, basic pharmacology, orders/labels/rights, routes, safety, allergies, immunizations, screening, storage, and patient teaching.

1. Which task is **within** the typical scope of a CMA related to medications?
   A. Prescribing a new antihypertensive drug
   B. Changing an insulin dose based on personal judgment
   C. Administering an ordered vaccine and documenting it according to policy
   D. Advising a patient to stop a medication prescribed by another provider
2. The **generic name** of a drug is best described as:
   A. The brand name chosen by a manufacturer
   B. The chemical formula

C. The official, nonproprietary name used across manufacturers
D. A nickname commonly used by patients

3. A complete medication order should include all of the following **except**:
   A. Patient's name
   B. Medication name
   C. Provider's favorite color
   D. Route and frequency
4. Before administering a medication, the CMA checks the patient's name and date of birth against the chart and the wristband. This action reflects which medication is "right"?
   A. Right route
   B. Right patient
   C. Right documentation
   D. Right time
5. A provider writes an order that is missing the route of administration. What is the **best** action for the CMA?
   A. Guess the most common route and proceed
   B. Ask another CMA what route to use
   C. Clarify the missing information with the provider before administering
   D. Leave the order blank and administer no medication
6. Which route of administration generally provides the **fastest** onset of action?
   A. Oral
   B. Intramuscular
   C. Intravenous
   D. Topical
7. A bottle of liquid medication is labeled "shake well before use." This likely indicates the medication is a:
   A. Tablet
   B. Capsule
   C. Suspension
   D. Suppository
8. Which of the following is the **safest** action when a dosage seems unusually high for a pediatric patient?
   A. Administer it as written to avoid delays
   B. Ask the parent if it seems right
   C. Double-check the order and calculations and consult the provider if there is doubt
   D. Give half the dose without clarification
9. High-alert medications are best described as drugs that:
   A. Are more expensive than others
   B. Always taste unpleasant
   C. Have a higher risk of causing serious harm if an error occurs
   D. Can be given without provider oversight
10. A patient states they are allergic to penicillin and previously developed hives after taking it. The CMA should:
    A. Document the allergy and avoid penicillin-class drugs without provider review
    B. Assume it was a side effect and proceed
    C. Decide the allergy is not real
    D. Ignore the allergy because it happened years ago
11. A patient reports stomach upset when taking a certain medication but no rash or breathing problems. This is

most likely:
A. A life-threatening allergy
B. A typical side effect rather than a true allergy
C. Not worth documenting
D. A reason to avoid all medications

12. When preparing to administer an intramuscular vaccine to an adult, the CMA should:
A. Select an appropriate IM site such as the deltoid according to policy
B. Inject into the forearm
C. Use any site the patient points to
D. Administer it orally instead

13. Which piece of information is **essential** to document after administering a vaccine?
A. Patient's favorite color
B. Date, vaccine name, lot number, manufacturer, dose, route, and site
C. Weather conditions
D. Provider's lunch choice

14. A vaccine has been left at room temperature all weekend instead of in the recommended refrigerator. The CMA should:
A. Use it quickly before it gets any warmer
B. Return it to the fridge and use it later
C. Follow policy, which typically includes discarding it and not using it on patients
D. Freeze it to "reset" the temperature

15. A patient scheduled for a vaccine reports a history of severe anaphylactic reaction to that same vaccine. What is the **best** action?
A. Administer it anyway but watch closely
B. Proceed if the patient insists
C. Do not administer and notify the provider immediately to review contraindications
D. Give a smaller dose instead

16. Screening before vaccination may include questions about:
A. Favorite hobbies
B. Current illness, previous reactions, and specific allergies
C. Preferred sports team
D. Shoe size

17. A patient asks, "Why are vaccines important if I feel healthy?" The CMA's **best** response is:
A. "They're required, so you just have to get them."
B. "Vaccines help your immune system prevent serious diseases, protecting you and people around you."
C. "They don't matter if you're healthy."
D. "They are only for very sick people."

18. After a vaccine, a patient asks what reactions to expect. Which response is most appropriate?
A. "You will definitely have a severe reaction."
B. "You might have mild soreness, redness, or a low-grade fever, but call us or seek care right away if you have trouble breathing or swelling of your face or throat."
C. "You won't feel anything at all."
D. "Don't call us about any reactions."

19. A patient is unsure how to take a new oral medication. The CMA should:

A. Tell them to take it however they want
B. Provide clear instructions according to the provider's order and label, and encourage questions
C. Refer them to internet forums only
D. Tell them to double the dose if they feel worse

20. Which action best reflects the **right documentation** in medication administration?
A. Writing "meds given" with no details
B. Documenting medication name, dose, route, time, site (if applicable), and any immediate patient response
C. Documenting medications before actually giving them
D. Leaving documentation for the end of the shift

21. A provider writes an order with an unclear abbreviation for dose. The CMA's **best** response is to:
A. Guess what the abbreviation means
B. Ask a patient what they usually take
C. Clarify the dose with the provider before preparation or administration
D. Ignore the abbreviation and skip the medication

22. A patient receiving a new medication reports feeling "strange" and lightheaded shortly after the dose. The CMA should:
A. Ignore it since they didn't specify details
B. Check vital signs and promptly notify the provider of the symptoms
C. Tell the patient it's just in their head
D. Advise them to drive home immediately

23. Which of the following is the **best** example of safe handling of a high-alert medication?
A. Administering it quickly without checking details
B. Double-checking the drug, dose, route, and patient identity per policy before administration
C. Letting patients measure their own dose in the office
D. Ignoring facility protocols to save time

24. A parent declines a recommended vaccine for their child. The CMA should:
A. Yell at the parent to comply
B. Respectfully provide accurate information, answer questions, and notify the provider
C. Give the vaccine anyway without telling them
D. Refuse future care to the family

25. A CMA recognizes that a near-miss medication error occurred (they caught the mistake before giving the drug). What is the appropriate action?
A. Say nothing since no harm occurred
B. Report the near miss according to policy so processes can be improved
C. Blame another staff member informally
D. Post about it anonymously online

Answer Key – Chapter 6 (with Justifications)

1. **C** – Administering an ordered vaccine and documenting it is within CMA scope under delegation; prescribing or changing doses independently is outside scope.
2. **C** – The generic name is the official nonproprietary name used across manufacturers, unlike brand names tied to specific companies.
3. **C** – Provider's favorite color is irrelevant; a complete order needs patient, medication, dose, route, frequency,

and provider authorization.

4. **B** – Verifying name and date of birth against records reflects the "right patient" medication safety check.
5. **C** – Missing route requires clarification from the provider; guessing a route is unsafe.
6. **C** – Intravenous medications generally have the fastest onset because they go directly into the bloodstream.
7. **C** – Suspensions contain particles that settle and must be shaken to distribute the medication evenly.
8. **C** – An unusually high pediatric dose should be double-checked and clarified with the provider, not given without question or arbitrarily altered.
9. **C** – High-alert medications are those where errors are more likely to cause serious harm, requiring extra caution.
10. **A** – A history of hives with penicillin suggests a true allergy; these should be documented, and such drugs avoided or reviewed carefully by the provider.
11. **B** – Stomach upset is more consistent with a typical side effect than a true allergy but should still be documented.
12. **A** – Intramuscular vaccines in adults are commonly given in the deltoid, following guidelines and policy.
13. **B** – Proper vaccine documentation includes date, name, lot number, manufacturer, dose, route, and site, supporting safety and tracking.
14. **C** – Vaccines stored outside recommended temperatures are generally considered compromised and should not be used; policy will guide disposal.
15. **C** – A history of severe anaphylaxis is a serious contraindication; the provider must review, and the vaccine should not be given without that review.
16. **B** – Screening questions focus on current illness, past reactions, and specific allergies relevant to vaccine safety.
17. **B** – This explanation emphasizes immune protection for both the individual and the community, which is a key vaccine benefit.
18. **B** – This response sets realistic expectations about mild reactions and clearly identifies serious symptoms that require urgent attention.
19. **B** – Clear instructions based on the order and label, plus encouraging questions, support safe medication use and adherence.
20. **B** – Right documentation includes all key details of what was given, how, when, where, and any immediate response.
21. **C** – Unclear abbreviations must be clarified with the provider to avoid dosing errors; guessing is unsafe.
22. **B** – New symptoms after a medication should be taken seriously; checking vitals and notifying the provider is appropriate.
23. **B** – High-alert medications should be double-checked carefully according to policy before administration to minimize risk.
24. **B** – Respectful education and provider involvement honor patient autonomy while promoting accurate information; secret administration or hostility is inappropriate.
25. **B** – Near misses should be reported to improve systems and prevent future errors, even though no harm occurred this time.

Chapter 7

Clinical Procedures and Diagnostic Testing

Clinical procedures and office-based diagnostic tests are a big part of a CMA's daily work. You might move from preparing patients for minor procedures to collecting specimens and running point-of-care (POC) tests all in the same hour. This chapter focuses on safe, accurate performance of common office procedures and diagnostic tests, and on how the CMA supports the provider throughout these processes.

7.1 The CMA's Role in Clinical Procedures and Testing

CMAS ARE OFTEN THE hands-on support team for clinical procedures and diagnostic tests in outpatient settings. You help prepare the environment, the patient, and the equipment, and you assist the provider before, during, and after procedures. The exam tests whether you understand your responsibilities and where your role stops.

- Preparing patients, equipment, and the environment
- Assisting during and after procedures within scope

Preparation includes checking that the room is stocked and clean, that equipment is functioning, and that supplies are ready and not expired. You also verify patient identity, explain what will happen in simple language, and obtain vital signs or baseline information as ordered. Positioning the patient appropriately and ensuring privacy with gowns or drapes are key steps. On exam questions, correct answers usually show the CMA anticipating needs and preparing carefully rather than rushing into a procedure unprepared.

Assisting during procedures might involve handing instruments, maintaining a clean or sterile field (within your training), and monitoring the patient for discomfort or signs of distress. Afterward, you may help apply dressings, provide post-procedure instructions, and clean and disinfect the room. You also document what happened, including patient tolerance and any specimens collected. The exam expects you to support the provider but not independently perform complex procedures that are beyond your scope.

7.2 Patient Identification, Verification, and Safety Checks

BEFORE ANY CLINICAL procedure or diagnostic test, confirming you have the right patient and right test is critical. Mistakes at this step can lead to wrong procedures, incorrect results, and serious harm. The exam frequently uses scenarios where a simple ID check could prevent an error.

- Verifying patient identity and procedure
- Confirming allergies and relevant history before procedures

Verifying identity typically involves using at least two identifiers, such as full name and date of birth, and comparing them to the chart or labels. You may also confirm the specific procedure or test being performed, especially if multiple tests are ordered. If something does not match, you must pause and clarify before proceeding. Exam questions often reward answers where the CMA stops a procedure when identifiers don't align instead of ignoring the discrepancy.

Confirming allergies and relevant history helps prevent complications during procedures or testing. For example, asking about latex allergies before using certain gloves or supplies, or checking for bleeding disorders before a venipuncture. You might also ask about medications that could affect results, like anticoagulants or fasting status. On the exam, skipping this step—especially when the scenario hints at allergy or risk—is usually the wrong choice; safe practice means screening and verifying before you begin.

7.3 Specimen Collection: Urine and Stool

URINE AND STOOL SPECIMENS are common in outpatient clinics and must be collected and handled carefully to ensure valid results. The CMA often provides instructions to patients, collects or receives specimens, and labels and prepares them for testing or transport. The exam tests both your technical and communication skills in these processes.

- Collecting and labeling urine specimens (including clean-catch)
- Handling stool specimens and patient instructions

Urine collection may involve random specimens, first-morning samples, timed collections, or clean-catch midstream specimens. Clean-catch procedures require specific steps to reduce contamination, such as cleansing the urethral area and collecting midstream urine after a small amount has been voided. Accurate labeling with patient name, date of birth, date/time, and test requested is essential, as is proper storage if not analyzed immediately. Exam questions often test whether you give clear, step-by-step instructions and label specimens before leaving the room or handing them off.

Stool specimens may be collected for occult blood testing, culture, or other purposes. You should instruct patients on how to collect the sample without contaminating it with urine or toilet water and how much to provide. Appropriate containers and tools (like spatulas or collection devices) must be used, and labeling is again critical. The exam will often present you with a specimen that was collected incorrectly or unlabeled and expect you to recognize that it must be rejected and recollected, not guessed about.

7.4 Specimen Collection: Blood and Capillary Testing

BLOOD SPECIMENS ARE central to many diagnostic tests, and CMAs may perform venipuncture and capillary sticks depending on training and state rules. Proper technique and safety are essential to protect both patients and staff. The exam focuses on identification, order of draw awareness, and complication prevention.

- Basic venipuncture and capillary collection principles
- Preventing complications such as hemolysis, fainting, or hematoma

Basic venipuncture principles include selecting an appropriate vein (often in the antecubital area), applying a tourniquet for the correct amount of time, cleansing the site, and inserting the needle at an appropriate angle. Tubes are filled in a recommended order of draw to avoid cross-contamination of additives. After collection, you release the tourniquet, withdraw the needle, apply pressure, and properly dispose of sharps. Exam questions frequently test whether you recognize steps done out of order or missed, such as failing to release the tourniquet.

Capillary collection (finger sticks or heel sticks) may be used for point-of-care tests like glucose or hemoglobin. Warmth, proper site selection, and avoiding "milking" the finger too aggressively help reduce hemolysis and discomfort. Patients may feel lightheaded or faint during blood collection, so observing them and being ready to assist is important. On the exam, safe answers often involve stopping the procedure if the patient says they feel faint, positioning them safely, and notifying the provider as needed.

7.5 Point-of-Care Testing (POCT) and Quality Control

POINT-OF-CARE TESTS (POCT) provide rapid results in the office, such as glucose checks, rapid strep tests, or urine dipsticks. While convenient, they must be performed and interpreted accurately. The exam expects you to understand quality control and basic test principles.

- Common POCT types and procedures
- Quality control checks and reagent handling

Common POCT includes blood glucose meters, rapid antigen tests (like strep or flu), urine dipstick analysis, and some hemoglobin or cholesterol tests. Each test has specific instructions for sample collection, timing, and interpretation, often including color change charts or digital readouts. You must follow manufacturer instructions closely and document results clearly. Exam questions often involve mis-timed readings or improper sample application as traps.

Quality control (QC) involves running control solutions or materials at specified intervals to verify that testing devices and reagents are working properly. Reagents and test strips must be stored correctly and used before their expiration dates. If QC results are out of range, patient testing must be halted until the issue is resolved. The exam frequently rewards answers where the CMA recognizes invalid QC and refuses to report patient results based on faulty tests.

7.6 Electrocardiography (ECG/EKG) Basics

ECGS (OR EKGS) RECORD the heart's electrical activity and are commonly performed in outpatient settings. CMAs often apply leads, run the tracing, and ensure the recording quality is acceptable. The exam expects basic familiarity with lead placement and artifact recognition, not advanced interpretation.

- Proper lead placement and patient preparation
- Recognizing and reducing artifact and interference

Correct lead placement includes placing limb leads on the arms and legs (or their equivalents, such as upper arms and lower legs) and chest (precordial) leads in specific intercostal spaces and positions. You should prepare the skin by cleaning and sometimes lightly abrading to improve conductivity. Explaining the procedure and asking the patient to lie still and relaxed helps reduce artifacts. Exam questions may show incorrect lead placement or ask how to improve a poor tracing.

Artifact can be caused by patient movement, muscle tension, loose electrodes, or external electrical interference. Common artifacts include wandering baselines, somatic tremor, and AC interference. To reduce them, you may reposition the patient, warm the room, secure leads, or move the ECG machine away from other equipment. The exam tends to favor answers where the CMA systematically checks and corrects possible causes of artifact rather than assuming the heart rhythm is abnormal based solely on a distorted tracing.

7.7 Respiratory and Pulmonary Function Testing

PULMONARY FUNCTION tests (PFTs) and peak flow measurements assess how well the lungs are working. CMAs may assist with or perform basic tests like spirometry or peak flow under supervision. The exam tests your understanding of patient coaching and accurate performance.

- Peak flow and basic spirometry procedures
- Coaching patients to obtain valid results

Peak flow meters measure how quickly air can be exhaled, often used in asthma management. You should instruct patients to stand or sit upright, take a deep breath, seal their lips tightly around the mouthpiece, and blow out as hard and fast as possible. The test is usually repeated several times, and the best effort is recorded. Exam questions may ask which coaching phrase will get the most accurate result.

Basic spirometry measures volumes and flows during inhalation and exhalation. Patients need clear instructions and practice attempts to perform the maneuvers correctly. You may need to demonstrate the technique and provide encouragement between attempts. Valid results depend on maximal effort and proper technique; half-hearted or improperly done efforts can give misleading readings. On the exam, responses that show you recognizing poor effort and re-coaching patients—as opposed to accepting obviously flawed tests—are typically correct.

7.8 Minor Office Procedures: Wound Care, Sutures, and Dressing Changes

MINOR OFFICE PROCEDURES can include wound care, suture removal, and dressing changes. CMAs often assist with these procedures under provider orders, helping maintain cleanliness, comfort, and safety. The exam focuses on aseptic technique, observation, and patient instructions.

- Assisting with wound care and dressing changes
- Suture and staple removal support within scope

Assisting with wound care involves preparing the area with clean or sterile supplies as ordered, handing instruments, and helping the provider assess the wound. You may help clean the wound with appropriate solutions and apply dressings using aseptic technique. Observing and reporting signs of infection—such as redness, warmth, swelling, increased pain, or drainage—is critical. Exam questions often present wound descriptions and ask what should be reported or how to maintain cleanliness during care.

Suture and staple removal may be performed by CMAs in some settings under provider orders and according to policy, using sterile instruments and careful technique. You must support the wound as needed, remove closures in a way that prevents tissue trauma, and apply steri-strips or dressings if ordered. After removal, you observe the wound edges for proper approximation and signs of dehiscence. The exam will likely emphasize knowing when to stop and notify the provider, such as if wound edges separate or significant bleeding occurs.

7.9 Gynecologic, Urologic, and Specialty Office Procedures

GYNECOLOGIC AND UROLOGIC procedures, as well as other specialty tests, are common in ambulatory care. CMAs help with preparation, positioning, and patient support, ensuring privacy and dignity. The exam tests whether you understand your role and maintain professionalism.

- Assisting with pelvic exams, Pap tests, and urologic procedures
- Providing emotional support and clear instructions during intimate procedures

For pelvic exams and Pap tests, you prepare the exam room with appropriate equipment, supplies, and drapes. You ensure the patient has privacy to undress, provide a gown, and explain what will happen and how they will be positioned (often lithotomy position for pelvic exams). During the procedure, you may hand instruments and label specimens. Exam questions often look for answers that emphasize privacy, respect, and accurate specimen handling.

Urologic procedures or tests might include catheterization, urinary flow tests, or prostate exams assisted by the provider. Your role can involve gathering supplies, positioning the patient, and explaining the process to reduce anxiety. Intimate procedures can be stressful, so offering reassurance, answering questions, and maintaining a calm, nonjudgmental demeanor is essential. The exam tends to favor responses where the CMA is sensitive to the patient's modesty and emotional comfort rather than being brusque or dismissive.

7.10 Documentation, Result Reporting, and Follow-Up

ACCURATE DOCUMENTATION and appropriate handling of test results are critical for patient safety and continuity of care. The CMA must record procedures and results correctly and follow protocols for reporting and follow-up. The exam tests whether you treat diagnostic information carefully and ethically.

- Documenting procedures, specimens, and test results clearly
- Reporting critical or abnormal results and ensuring follow-up

Documentation should include the name of the procedure or test, date and time, site (if applicable), patient tolerance, and any specimens collected (with identifiers). For POCT, you document the result, units, and any immediate actions taken. If a specimen is sent to a lab, you ensure requisition forms are accurate and match labels. Exam questions often show incomplete or vague documentation and expect you to choose more precise entries.

Reporting critical or abnormal results usually follows a specific protocol, such as notifying the provider immediately and documenting whom you notified and when. You should not interpret results independently or give diagnoses, but you can inform patients that the provider will review and discuss findings. Ensuring follow-up might include scheduling additional tests, visits, or reinforcing that the provider will call with results. On the exam, answers that involve ignoring abnormal results or sharing them casually without provider input are typically unsafe and incorrect.

Practice Questions – Chapter 7 (25 Questions)

THESE QUESTIONS ARE tied to Chapter 7: clinical procedures, patient verification, specimens, POCT, EKG, pulmonary tests, minor procedures, intimate exams, documentation, and result handling.

1. Before performing a wound dressing change, the CMA's **first** priority is to:
   A. Open all sterile packages
   B. Confirm patient identity and verify the correct procedure
   C. Ask the patient about their occupation
   D. Call the lab
2. Which action best demonstrates proper **patient identification** before a diagnostic test?
   A. Asking, "Are you John?" and accepting "yes"

B. Calling the patient by first name only
C. Asking the patient to state their full name and date of birth and comparing to the chart
D. Identifying the patient based on how they look

3. A patient with a known latex allergy is scheduled for a minor procedure. What is the **best** CMA response?
A. Use latex gloves anyway but work quickly
B. Inform the provider and ensure latex-free supplies are used
C. Cancel the procedure without telling anyone
D. Ignore the allergy if no rash is visible

4. Which instruction is appropriate for a **clean-catch midstream urine** sample?
A. "Void directly into the container as soon as you start urinating."
B. "Clean the area as instructed, start urinating into the toilet, then collect the midstream urine in the container."
C. "Collect only the first few drops of urine."
D. "No cleaning is necessary before collecting."

5. A urine specimen is handed to the CMA with no label on the container. The CMA should:
A. Guess which patient it belongs to based on schedule
B. Label it using the name on the collection cup
C. Discard the specimen per policy and request a new, properly labeled sample
D. Send it to the lab and let them figure it out

6. During venipuncture, the patient says they feel dizzy and lightheaded. The CMA's **priority** is to:
A. Continue drawing blood to finish quickly
B. Stop the procedure, release the tourniquet, remove the needle, and assist the patient to a safe position
C. Ignore the complaint
D. Ask the patient to stand up

7. Which action can help prevent **hemolysis** in a blood specimen?
A. Vigorously shaking the tube
B. Using a needle that is too small
C. Gently inverting tubes according to instructions rather than shaking
D. Drawing blood through a very long, narrow catheter

8. When performing POCT with a glucose meter, the CMA should:
A. Use the device even if quality control (QC) results are out of range
B. Document results only if they seem normal
C. Follow manufacturer instructions, run QC as scheduled, and not use the device if QC fails
D. Let patients perform their own tests unsupervised

9. A rapid strep test requires reading the result in exactly 5 minutes. Reading it at 15 minutes may:
A. Have no impact on accuracy
B. Increase accuracy
C. Produce false results because the test is not validated for that time
D. Automatically cancel the test

10. When placing ECG chest (precordial) leads, the CMA should:
A. Place them anywhere on the chest as long as they stick
B. Follow standard anatomical landmarks for each lead position
C. Put all chest leads on the left side only
D. Place them over clothing for comfort

11. An ECG tracing shows a lot of jagged lines that correspond to patient shivering. This artifact is most likely due to:
    A. Loose paper in the machine
    B. Somatic tremor from muscle movement
    C. AC interference from power lines
    D. A heart attack
12. Which instruction will most help a patient produce a valid **peak flow** reading?
    A. "Take a normal breath and blow out gently."
    B. "Take a deep breath, seal your lips around the mouthpiece, and blow out as hard and fast as you can."
    C. "Whisper into the device slowly."
    D. "Cough into it repeatedly."
13. During a dressing change, the CMA notices increased redness, warmth, swelling, and yellow drainage at the wound site. The **best** action is to:
    A. Document findings and notify the provider of possible infection signs
    B. Ignore it; this is always normal
    C. Clean it quickly without telling anyone
    D. Remove all stitches immediately
14. When assisting with suture removal under provider order, the CMA should:
    A. Pull knots through the tissue
    B. Use sterile instruments and cut sutures close to the skin before gently pulling them out
    C. Yank all sutures out quickly to reduce discomfort
    D. Remove sutures even if the wound edges are open and gaping
15. Before a pelvic exam, the CMA's actions should include:
    A. Leaving the door open for ventilation
    B. Providing a gown and drape, explaining the procedure, and ensuring privacy
    C. Having the patient remain fully dressed
    D. Making jokes about the exam to lighten the mood
16. During an intimate procedure, a patient appears very anxious and tearful. The CMA should:
    A. Ignore the emotions and proceed
    B. Stop the procedure permanently
    C. Acknowledge their feelings, explain each step calmly, and offer to pause or involve a support person if appropriate
    D. Tell them to "relax and get over it"
17. A patient asks the CMA to explain detailed ECG results and whether they have heart disease. The **best** CMA response is:
    A. "Yes, you definitely have heart disease."
    B. "No, you're perfectly fine."
    C. "The provider will review your ECG and discuss the results with you; I'll let them know you have questions."
    D. "Let's guess based on the lines."
18. A specimen for a throat culture must be sent to an external lab. The CMA should:
    A. Place the swab in any available container
    B. Label the specimen properly, complete the requisition form, and follow transport instructions
    C. Leave it on the counter until the end of the day

D. Ask the patient to deliver it themselves without labeling

19. After performing a rapid POCT, the CMA forgets to document the result immediately. Later, they can't recall the exact value and guess. This is:
    A. Acceptable if the guess is close
    B. An example of falsifying documentation and unsafe practice
    C. Encouraged to save time
    D. Required when busy
20. A critical lab result is phoned to the clinic, indicating dangerously high potassium. The CMA receiving the call should:
    A. Take the message casually and call back later
    B. Document the result, read back the value to verify, and immediately notify the provider according to policy
    C. Tell the lab it can wait until tomorrow
    D. Share the result with other patients as an example
21. When charting a procedure, which entry is most appropriate?
    A. "Stuff done, patient okay."
    B. "Wound care performed."
    C. "Dressing change performed to left forearm laceration at 10:15; wound cleansed with normal saline; sterile dressing applied; patient tolerated well."
    D. "Look at the wound; it seems fine."
22. A patient refuses to complete a recommended diagnostic test. The CMA should:
    A. Force the patient to do it
    B. Respect the refusal, document it, and notify the provider
    C. Mark the test as completed anyway
    D. Argue loudly until the patient agrees
23. A POCT urine dipstick shows abnormal findings. The CMA should:
    A. Ignore abnormalities and file results
    B. Document the results clearly and notify the provider for interpretation
    C. Diagnose a urinary tract infection
    D. Throw away the strip without telling anyone
24. When a patient's test result is available, the CMA's role typically includes:
    A. Interpreting the result and giving a diagnosis
    B. Ensuring the result is entered in the record and letting the provider know so they can discuss it with the patient
    C. Hiding abnormal results
    D. Posting results on social media
25. A patient's ECG shows heavy artifacts and is unreadable. The CMA's **best** action is to:
    A. Label it as normal and file it
    B. Repeat the ECG after checking lead placement and instructing the patient to remain still
    C. Throw away the tracing and do nothing
    D. Assume the artifact is a heart attack

Answer Key – Chapter 7 (with Justifications)

1. **B** – Confirming patient identity and procedure is the first priority to prevent wrong-patient or wrong-

procedure errors.

2. **C** – Having the patient state full name and date of birth and comparing to the chart ensures accurate identification; appearance alone is unreliable.
3. **B** – Latex allergy must be taken seriously; informing the provider and using latex-free supplies protects patient safety.
4. **B** – Clean-catch midstream collection requires cleansing, discarding the initial urine, and collecting midstream to reduce contamination.
5. **C** – Unlabeled specimens cannot be safely matched to a patient; they must be discarded per policy and recollected to ensure accuracy.
6. **B** – Dizziness during venipuncture signals potential fainting; the CMA must stop, release the tourniquet, remove the needle, and ensure patient safety.
7. **C** – Gentle inversion of tubes according to instructions helps mix additives without damaging cells; vigorous shaking and tiny needles increase hemolysis risk.
8. **C** – POCT devices should not be used when QC is out of range; following instructions and halting testing when QC fails ensures reliability.
9. **C** – Reading tests outside the validated time frame can produce false results; timing is critical for accuracy.
10. **B** – Chest leads must be placed at specific anatomical landmarks to obtain a valid ECG; random or over-clothing placement is incorrect.
11. **B** – Jagged lines from shivering indicate somatic tremor artifacts due to muscle movement, not heart pathology itself.
12. **B** – A deep breath followed by a hard, fast exhalation is necessary for a valid peak flow reading.
13. **A** – Increased redness, warmth, swelling, and yellow drainage suggest infection and should be documented and reported to the provider.
14. **B** – Sterile instruments and cutting sutures near the skin before gently pulling them out help prevent tissue trauma; open or gaping wounds require provider review.
15. **B** – Providing a gown and drape, explaining, and ensuring privacy preserve dignity and comfort during pelvic exams.
16. **C** – Acknowledging feelings, explaining steps, and offering to pause or involve support are appropriate responses to anxiety during intimate procedures.
17. **C** – The CMA must stay within scope, deferring ECG interpretation and diagnosis to the provider while ensuring the provider knows the patient has questions.
18. **B** – Proper labeling, requisition completion, and following transport instructions are essential for valid lab processing.
19. **B** – Guessing results after forgetting them is falsification and unsafe; accurate, timely documentation is mandatory.
20. **B** – Critical results require immediate documentation, read-back verification, and prompt provider notification per policy.
21. **C** – This entry clearly describes what was done, where, when, and how the patient tolerated it, supporting continuity and legal documentation.
22. **B** – Patients may refuse tests; the CMA should document the refusal and notify the provider, not force or falsify.
23. **B** – Abnormal POCT findings must be documented and brought to the provider for interpretation; the CMA does not diagnose.
24. **B** – The CMA ensures results are in the record and alerts the provider, who is responsible for interpretation

and discussion with the patient.

25. **B** – Heavy artifact requires correcting lead placement and patient movement and repeating the ECG; labeling it as normal or assuming a heart attack is unsafe.

Chapter 8

Minor Office Surgery and Emergency Preparedness

Outpatient clinics handle a surprising amount of minor surgery and urgent issues. As a CMA, you're often the one setting up sterile fields, assisting providers, and responding when patients suddenly feel faint or show emergency symptoms. This chapter covers your role in minor office surgical procedures and how you help prepare for and respond to emergencies safely and within your scope.

8.1 The CMA's Role in Minor Office Surgery

MINOR OFFICE SURGERY includes procedures like lesion removal, biopsies, and incision and drainage. The CMA is often the main assistant, making sure the room, equipment, and patient are ready. The exam tests whether you know how to support these procedures without stepping outside your scope.

- Preparing the room, equipment, and patient
- Assisting during the procedure and supporting recovery

Preparing for minor surgery includes checking that the procedure room is clean, stocked, and organized. You verify that instruments are sterile, supplies are not expired, and equipment like lights or cautery units are working. You also confirm patient identity, explain what will happen in simple terms, and ensure informed consent has been documented by the provider. On exam questions, correct answers often show the CMA checking all of these basics rather than jumping straight into the procedure.

Assisting during the procedure may involve positioning the patient, handing instruments, managing supplies, and observing for signs of discomfort or distress. You help maintain a clean or sterile field as ordered and respond quickly when the provider requests tools or materials. After the procedure, you may assist with the dressing application, help the patient sit up slowly, and provide immediate post-procedure instructions. The exam favors answers where the CMA remains attentive, safety-focused, and careful about observation and documentation.

8.2 Maintaining Sterile Fields and Aseptic Technique

STERILE TECHNIQUE IS critical during minor surgical procedures to reduce infection risk. The CMA plays a major role in maintaining the sterile field and recognizing contamination. The exam frequently uses "sterile field" questions to see whether you know what breaks sterility and what to do when that happens.

- Principles of a sterile field
- Recognizing and responding to breaks in sterility

Sterile fields include only sterile items, and sterile objects should only touch other sterile objects. Non-sterile items must stay outside the field, and you must avoid reaching over the sterile area or turning your back on it. Sterile packages must be opened carefully so their contents can drop onto the field without touching non-sterile surfaces. Exam questions often describe subtle mistakes—like a sleeve brushing the field—that should trigger restarting or replacing contaminated items.

Recognizing a break in sterility means paying attention to touching, positioning, and movements during a procedure. If an instrument falls below waist level, touches an unsterile surface, or is uncertain in its sterility, it must be considered contaminated. The correct response is to remove the contaminated item and replace it with a sterile one, and to speak up even if it feels awkward. On the exam, ignoring a suspected contamination to "save time" is almost always the wrong answer.

8.3 Instrument Handling and Minor Surgical Sets

MINOR SURGERY USES specific instruments—like forceps, scissors, scalpels, and needle holders—that must be handled correctly. The CMA is expected to recognize common instruments and pass them safely to the provider. The exam often tests your understanding of safe handling rather than memorizing every instrument by name.

- Safe handling and passing of instruments
- Basic awareness of common minor surgical instruments

Safe handling involves grasping instruments in a way that avoids injury to you or the provider. Sharps, such as scalpels or suture needles, should be passed handle-first with a clear verbal cue if needed. You should know how to place used instruments in designated trays without tossing or stacking them dangerously. On exam scenarios, correct answers show attentive handling and awareness of sharps safety within the sterile field.

Common minor surgical instruments can include hemostats for clamping, scissors for cutting tissue or sutures, forceps for grasping, and needle holders for suturing. While you may not need to name every type, recognizing categories and general uses is helpful. For example, using bandage scissors instead of delicate tissue scissors would be inappropriate. The exam may describe an instrument by function ("used to grasp tissue") and expect you to identify safe use or correct selection in a given scenario.

8.4 Local Anesthesia and Patient Monitoring

LOCAL ANESTHESIA NUMBS a specific area so minor surgery can be performed without significant pain. Although CMAs do not independently administer anesthetics, you often assist and monitor patients during their use. The exam checks if you understand what to watch for and how to respond.

- Supporting local anesthesia administration
- Monitoring for adverse reactions and patient comfort

Supporting local anesthesia may involve preparing the area, laying out the medication and supplies, and confirming the correct patient and site. You may help position the patient and reassure them as the injection is given. It's important to note where and how much anesthetic is used, as documented by the provider. On test questions, the CMA should never decide which anesthetic to use or how much; that responsibility lies with the provider.

Monitoring after local anesthesia includes watching for signs of allergic reaction, such as rash, itching, or difficulty breathing, as well as systemic symptoms like dizziness or altered consciousness. You also check that the area is adequately numb before the procedure progresses too far and ask the patient about their comfort level. If a patient reports chest pain, shortness of breath, or feels faint, you must act immediately to ensure safety and notify the provider. Exam answers typically reward prompt recognition and escalation of concerning signs rather than dismissing them.

8.5 Surgical Site Preparation, Draping, and Post-Procedure Dressing

PREPARING THE SURGICAL site and using drapes correctly helps reduce infection and protect patient privacy. After the procedure, dressings must be applied and secured to protect the wound. The CMA often assists with all of these steps.

- Skin preparation and draping techniques
- Applying and securing dressings after minor surgery

Skin preparation usually involves cleansing the area with an antiseptic solution using outward circular motions from the center, avoiding re-contaminating prepared skin. Hair may be clipped, not shaved, if needed for access. Drapes are placed to expose only the surgical area while covering other skin and maintaining modesty. Exam questions often ask about the correct direction of skin prep or whether a contaminated prep applicator can be reused (it cannot).

Applying dressings after the procedure involves using sterile or clean materials as ordered, covering the site fully, and securing with tape or bandages without excessive tension. You must avoid touching the inside of dressings that will contact the wound. Instructions may include how long to keep the dressing in place and how to care for the site at home. On the exam, safe answers show careful dressing technique and clear patient education about keeping the site clean and dry and watching for signs of infection.

8.6 Emergency Preparedness: Roles and Responsibilities

EVERY CLINIC MUST BE ready for emergencies, from fainting episodes to severe allergic reactions or cardiac arrest. The CMA plays an important role in recognizing emergencies, acting quickly, and supporting the team. The exam tests your understanding of your responsibilities in these high-stress moments.

- Recognizing common in-office emergencies
- Understanding your role in emergency response plans

Common emergencies include syncope (fainting), chest pain, difficulty breathing, seizures, severe allergic reactions, and injuries like falls. You may be the first person to see signs of distress, such as a patient becoming pale, sweaty, or unresponsive. Early recognition and rapid action can save lives. On the exam, any signs of chest pain, stroke symptoms, or anaphylaxis must be treated as emergencies, not routine complaints.

Your role in emergency response typically includes calling for help, activating emergency medical services (EMS) if instructed, retrieving emergency equipment, and performing basic life support within your training (like CPR) if necessary. You must also help clear areas, support documentation, and follow the clinic's emergency protocols. Exam questions favor answers where the CMA follows established plans and works as part of a team, rather than acting independently in ways that exceed training or delay definitive care.

8.7 Basic Life Support (BLS) Concepts and AED Use

BASIC LIFE SUPPORT (BLS) and AED (automated external defibrillator) use are critical skills in sudden cardiac emergencies. While the CMA exam won't replace BLS certification training, it does expect conceptual knowledge of your role. You should know what steps to take if a patient collapses.

- Recognizing cardiac arrest and initiating basic life support
- AED awareness and support role

Recognizing cardiac arrest means identifying unresponsiveness and abnormal or absent breathing. The immediate response is to call for help, start CPR if trained and allowed, and have someone retrieve the AED. Compressions should begin quickly with minimal interruptions while advanced help is summoned. On exam questions, the emphasis is on starting the chain of survival rather than checking a pulse for a long time or waiting for the provider.

AED awareness includes knowing where the device is stored, how to retrieve it quickly, and how to follow its prompts. While some CMAs may place pads and operate the AED, you must always follow your training and local regulations. The device itself analyzes the rhythm and gives voice prompts about when to deliver a shock and when to resume compressions. Test questions usually reward actions that prioritize early activation of EMS and AED use and continued CPR, not delaying to perform extensive assessments beyond your scope.

8.8 Managing Syncope, Seizures, and Acute Reactions

SYNCOPE (FAINTING), seizures, and acute reactions such as anaphylaxis can all occur in outpatient settings. The CMA must respond calmly and appropriately to protect the patient from further harm. The exam often includes these scenarios to test emergency thinking.

- Handling syncope and near-syncope in the office
- Responding to seizures and suspected anaphylaxis

For syncope or near-syncope, you should help the patient into a safe position—lying down or sitting with legs elevated—so blood flow to the brain improves. You monitor vital signs, loosen tight clothing, and ensure the patient doesn't fall or injure themselves. Once they recover, you should not simply send them home; the provider must evaluate them and decide on next steps. Exam answers that involve leaving a faint patient upright or alone are unsafe.

Seizure response includes protecting the patient from injury by clearing nearby objects and cushioning the head if possible, without restraining or placing anything in the mouth. After the seizure, you monitor breathing and position the patient in the recovery position if appropriate. Suspected anaphylaxis (severe allergic reaction) requires urgent action: notify the provider immediately, activate emergency protocols, and prepare emergency medications and equipment as instructed. On the exam, delaying action in anaphylaxis scenarios is almost always incorrect; rapid response is critical.

8.9 Emergency Drugs, Equipment, and Crash Carts (Awareness-Level)

MOST CLINICS MAINTAIN emergency drugs and equipment, often organized in a crash cart or emergency kit. CMAs are not expected to choose drug therapies but should know where emergency supplies are and how to help access them. The exam tests awareness rather than full pharmacologic detail.

- Awareness of common emergency supplies and drugs
- Maintaining readiness of emergency equipment

Common emergency supplies include oxygen delivery devices, bag-valve masks, suction equipment, IV supplies, and AEDs. Emergency drugs might include epinephrine, antihistamines, glucose, and others determined by the clinic and providers. You should know the location of these items and how to bring them quickly to the provider when needed. Exam questions may ask what you should do first when an emergency is declared, often involving retrieving the crash cart or AED and calling for help.

Maintaining readiness includes checking that equipment is present, functional, and within expiration dates according to facility schedules. This may involve verifying oxygen tank levels, confirming the AED is powered and showing readiness indicators, and checking drug expiration dates. If you notice missing or expired items, you must report and correct this before an emergency occurs. On the exam, ignoring missing or expired emergency supplies is considered unsafe practice.

8.10 Patient Education After Minor Surgery and Emergency Events

AFTER MINOR SURGERY or urgent events, patients need clear, simple instructions about what to do at home and when to seek further care. The CMA often provides or reinforces this education. The exam includes questions about what you should teach and how.

- Teaching wound care, activity limits, and warning signs after minor procedures
- Explaining follow-up and when to seek urgent help after emergency symptoms

Post-procedure education may include how to care for the wound (keeping it clean and dry), when to change dressings, and whether to avoid certain activities. You should explain normal expectations such as mild soreness or slight bruising, and abnormal signs such as increasing pain, redness, swelling, drainage, or fever. Written instructions are helpful, especially if the patient is anxious or has a lot to remember. On exam questions, teaching that is specific and emphasizes infection signs is generally correct.

After emergency symptoms—like a fainting episode, chest pain, or a seizure—patients and families may feel uncertain or scared. You should reinforce any provider instructions, explain any scheduled follow-up visits or tests, and clearly state when they should call the clinic or go to the emergency department. For example, chest pain, increasing shortness of breath, or new neurological symptoms should never be ignored. The exam rewards education that both empowers patients and encourages them to seek help promptly for serious warning signs.

Practice Questions – Chapter 8 (25 Questions)

THESE QUESTIONS ARE tied to Chapter 8: minor surgery prep, sterile fields, instruments, anesthesia support, site prep and dressings, emergency response, BLS/AED concepts, syncope/seizures/anaphylaxis, emergency equipment, and post-event teaching.

1. Before a minor surgical procedure, the CMA's **first** priority is to:
   A. Open all sterile supplies immediately
   B. Confirm patient identity, procedure, and consent status
   C. Ask about the patient's favorite TV show
   D. Turn off the exam room lights
2. Which action **violates** sterile field principles?
   A. Keeping sterile items above waist level

B. Avoiding reaching over the sterile field
C. Turning your back on the sterile field and then returning
D. Opening sterile packages so contents drop onto the field

3. During a procedure, a sterile instrument falls below waist level onto a non-sterile surface. The CMA should:
A. Pick it up and continue using it
B. Rinse it with tap water and reuse
C. Consider it contaminated and replace it with a sterile instrument
D. Wipe it with gauze and continue
4. A provider requests a sharp instrument. The **safest** way for the CMA to pass it is to:
A. Toss it gently toward the provider
B. Hand it blade-first for quick access
C. Pass it handle-first, ensuring both parties have a secure grip
D. Place it on the patient and let the provider pick it up
5. Which task related to local anesthesia is appropriate for the CMA?
A. Choosing which anesthetic and dose to use
B. Administering anesthesia without provider orders
C. Preparing supplies and monitoring the patient for reactions after the provider administers it
D. Instructing the provider on how much to inject
6. After local anesthesia is injected, a patient suddenly becomes dizzy and complains of difficulty breathing. The CMA should:
A. Assume it is normal and continue
B. Stop the procedure, call for the provider, and be prepared to assist with emergency measures
C. Tell the patient to breathe more slowly and ignore symptoms
D. Leave the room to avoid stress
7. Proper skin prep for a minor surgical site typically involves:
A. Scrubbing in small circles from the outer area inward
B. Using an antiseptic in outward circles from the center of the site
C. Using only plain water
D. Applying lotion to keep skin moist
8. Which dressing application is most appropriate after a minor surgical procedure?
A. Touching the inside of the dressing with bare hands before applying
B. Covering the wound with sterile materials and securing them without excessive tension
C. Leaving the wound completely open to air with no covering
D. Using tape directly on fresh sutures
9. A patient suddenly collapses in the waiting room and is unresponsive. The CMA's **first** action should be to:
A. Check responsiveness and breathing, then call for help and activate emergency response
B. Look for their insurance card
C. Move all chairs around before doing anything
D. Wait to see if the patient wakes up on their own
10. Recognizing cardiac arrest involves:
A. The patient being sleepy but responsive
B. The patient being unresponsive with abnormal or absent breathing
C. The patient complaining of headache
D. The patient hyperventilating but responsive

11. When an AED is brought to an unresponsive patient, the CMA should:
    A. Ignore the AED and wait for the provider
    B. Turn on the AED and follow its prompts within their training
    C. Use the AED only if the patient is awake
    D. Reprogram the AED before each use
12. During venipuncture, a patient faints. After assisting them to a safe position, the CMA should:
    A. Leave them alone to rest
    B. Monitor vital signs and notify the provider for evaluation
    C. Immediately discharge them from the clinic
    D. Ask them to stand up quickly to see if they faint again
13. When managing a seizure in the clinic, the CMA should:
    A. Try to hold the patient down and restrain movement
    B. Place an object in the patient's mouth to prevent biting the tongue
    C. Clear nearby objects to prevent injury and monitor until the seizure ends
    D. Shake the patient to stop the seizure
14. A patient receiving an injection develops hives, swelling around the mouth, and difficulty breathing. This scenario suggests:
    A. Mild anxiety only
    B. Anaphylaxis requiring immediate emergency response
    C. A normal reaction to all injections
    D. Simple dehydration
15. In suspected anaphylaxis, the CMA's **most appropriate** action is to:
    A. Reassure the patient and schedule a follow-up visit
    B. Immediately initiate emergency protocols, notify the provider, and prepare emergency medications and equipment as directed
    C. Offer the patient water
    D. Ignore symptoms and see the next patient
16. The purpose of a crash cart or emergency kit is to:
    A. Store personal items
    B. Provide quick access to emergency drugs and equipment in one organized place
    C. Keep everyday office supplies
    D. Display decorations
17. The CMA notices the AED's indicator shows a low battery. The **best** response is to:
    A. Ignore it until the next emergency
    B. Turn the AED off permanently
    C. Report and arrange for battery replacement according to policy
    D. Hide the AED so no one uses it
18. After a syncope episode, patient teaching should include:
    A. "This is always harmless; you don't need to worry."
    B. "Follow the provider's instructions, and report any future episodes, chest pain, or worsening symptoms immediately."
    C. "Don't tell anyone else about this."
    D. "You must avoid all activity forever."
19. Which statement is appropriate post-procedure wound care teaching?

A. "Leave the dressing on indefinitely."
B. "Keep the area clean and dry, change dressings as instructed, and call if you notice increasing redness, swelling, pain, or drainage."
C. "You can scratch or pick at the wound to help it heal."
D. "Soak the wound in dirty water to toughen it up."

20. After a minor office procedure, a patient asks when they should seek urgent care. The **best** CMA response is:
A. "Never; everything will be fine."
B. "Seek urgent care if you develop high fever, severe pain, heavy bleeding, or trouble breathing, or if the provider advised it."
C. "Only call if the dressing falls off."
D. "Don't contact us again; it's your problem now."
21. A CMA finds that epinephrine in the emergency kit expired last month. The appropriate action is to:
A. Ignore it since emergencies are rare
B. Replace it according to policy and report the issue so stock checks can be improved
C. Use it first to avoid waste
D. Disguise the expiration date
22. During a minor procedure, the CMA notices the provider's glove tears. The **best** response is to:
A. Ignore it and continue
B. Quietly leave the room
C. Inform the provider so they can change gloves and maintain infection control
D. Only change your own gloves
23. A patient is extremely anxious before a minor surgery and says, "I'm really scared something will go wrong." The CMA should respond by:
A. "You're overreacting; it's minor."
B. "You agreed to this, so you shouldn't be scared."
C. "It's understandable to feel nervous. Let me explain what will happen and what we do to keep you safe, and I'll stay with you."
D. "If you're scared, we should cancel everything immediately."
24. After performing a wound dressing change, the CMA documents: "Dressing changed." This entry is:
A. Complete and sufficient
B. Too detailed
C. Incomplete; documentation should include site, time, care provided, and patient tolerance
D. Unnecessary
25. A patient treated in the clinic for chest pain is sent to the emergency department by EMS. Later, the patient calls asking about their ED results. The CMA should:
A. Provide a full interpretation based on guesswork
B. Tell them to get results from the internet
C. Explain that the provider will review any available records and discuss results with them, and help schedule follow-up if needed
D. Refuse to speak with them

Answer Key – Chapter 8 (with Justifications)

1. **B** – Confirming patient identity, procedure, and consent ensures the right procedure is done on the right

patient and meets legal/ethical standards.

2. **C** – Turning your back on a sterile field and then returning is considered a break in sterility because you can no longer guarantee it was not contaminated.
3. **C** – Once a sterile instrument falls below waist level or touches a non-sterile surface, it must be considered contaminated and replaced.
4. **C** – Passing sharps handle-first with clear control minimizes risk of injury to both the CMA and provider.
5. **C** – The CMA may prepare supplies and monitor patients but cannot independently choose or administer local anesthetics without provider direction.
6. **B** – Dizziness and difficulty breathing after anesthesia may signal a serious reaction; the CMA must stop the procedure, call the provider, and be ready for emergency measures.
7. **B** – Proper skin prep typically uses antiseptic applied in outward circles from the center to move contaminants away from the incision site.
8. **B** – Sterile dressings should cover the wound fully and be secured without excessive tension that could impair circulation or disrupt closure.
9. **A** – Assessing responsiveness and breathing, then calling for help and activating emergency response is the correct first step for a collapse.
10. **B** – Cardiac arrest is characterized by unresponsiveness and absent or abnormal breathing, not just sleepiness or headache.
11. **B** – The AED should be turned on and its prompts followed as soon as it's available, consistent with training and protocols.
12. **B** – After syncope, monitoring vitals and notifying the provider ensures appropriate evaluation; leaving the patient alone is unsafe.
13. **C** – Clearing objects and monitoring the patient, without restraining or placing items in the mouth, is safe management of a seizure.
14. **B** – Hives, facial swelling, and difficulty breathing after an injection strongly suggest anaphylaxis, a life-threatening emergency.
15. **B** – Immediate emergency protocols, provider notification, and preparation of emergency meds/equipment are essential in suspected anaphylaxis.
16. **B** – A crash cart organizes emergency drugs and equipment for rapid access in urgent situations.
17. **C** – Low battery indicators must be addressed; arranging prompt replacement ensures AED readiness.
18. **B** – Teaching should reinforce provider instructions and emphasize reporting future episodes or serious symptoms promptly.
19. **B** – Proper teaching includes wound care steps and warning signs like increased redness, swelling, pain, or drainage.
20. **B** – Patients should seek urgent care for serious signs such as high fever, severe pain, heavy bleeding, or breathing problems, consistent with provider guidance.
21. **B** – Expired epinephrine is a safety issue; it must be replaced and the problem reported to improve stock management.
22. **C** – A torn glove compromises infection control; the provider must change gloves to protect both patient and provider.
23. **C** – Acknowledging fear and explaining safety measures while offering support is therapeutic and maintains professionalism.
24. **C** – "Dressing changed" is incomplete; documentation should specify location, time, care given, and patient tolerance for legal and clinical clarity.

25. **C** – The CMA should defer interpretation to the provider, explain that the provider will review records, and assist with arranging follow-up, staying within scope.

Chapter 9

Special Populations: Pediatrics, Geriatrics, and Obstetrics

Some patients need different approaches because of their age, life stage, or health changes. Pediatrics, geriatrics, and obstetric patients bring unique physical, emotional, and communication needs to each visit. This chapter focuses on how the CMA adapts assessments, communication, and safety practices for these special populations while staying within scope.

9.1 Caring for Pediatric Patients: General Principles

PEDIATRIC VISITS OFTEN involve not just the child but also parents or caregivers who have their own questions and concerns. Children may feel anxious, scared, or shy in the medical setting. The CMA must approach them with patience, clarity, and sensitivity.

- Building rapport and trust with children
- Involving parents and caregivers appropriately

Building rapport with children usually means getting down to their eye level, using a calm and friendly tone, and sometimes engaging in brief age-appropriate conversation before jumping into procedures. You might show them your stethoscope, demonstrate on a doll, or let them touch safe equipment to reduce fear. Avoiding sudden movements and explaining what you're doing in simple, non-threatening terms helps them feel more secure. On exam questions, answers that show the CMA being gentle, patient, and child-focused tend to be correct.

Involving parents or caregivers is essential, especially for younger children who can't fully understand or communicate on their own. You should include the adult in explanations, ask about the child's usual behavior and any concerns, and respect their role as decision-makers. At the same time, it's important to address the child directly when possible, so they don't feel ignored. The exam rewards approaches where the CMA balances caregiver involvement with respect for the child's voice and comfort.

9.2 Pediatric Development and Communication by Age

CHILDREN'S COMMUNICATION abilities and understanding change dramatically as they grow. A one-size-fits-all approach doesn't work well and can make visits harder than they need to be. The CMA should adjust language and expectations based on developmental stages.

- Communicating with infants and young children
- Communicating with school-age children and adolescents

With infants and toddlers, communication is mainly through tone of voice, facial expressions, and gentle touch. Comforting behaviors like speaking softly, smiling, and allowing a parent to hold the child when possible can reduce distress. For toddlers and preschoolers, simple, concrete explanations ("I'm going to listen to your heart" rather than "auscultate your chest") work best, and offering simple choices ("Which arm should we use?") can provide a sense of control. Exam questions typically favor responses that are developmentally appropriate and calm.

School-age children can usually understand more detailed explanations and may ask many questions. You can describe what you're doing in more detail and encourage them to participate, such as by holding a thermometer or counting heartbeats. Adolescents may value privacy and autonomy and might want to ask questions without parents present, especially about sensitive topics. The exam often tests whether you respect adolescent confidentiality within legal limits and speak with them respectfully, not as if they were small children.

9.3 Pediatric Vital Signs, Growth, and Safety

PEDIATRIC VITAL SIGNS and growth patterns differ from adults, and normal ranges vary by age. Safety, including preventing falls and injuries in the clinic, is especially important with children. The CMA must be aware of these differences when assessing and caring for pediatric patients.

- Age-based differences in vital signs and growth
- Ensuring safety and supervision in the clinic

Infants and young children usually have higher heart and respiratory rates and lower blood pressure than adults. Growth is tracked using standardized growth charts, with weight, length/height, and head circumference (for infants) plotted over time. Sudden jumps or drops in percentiles may signal a problem and should be reported to the provider. On exam questions, recognizing what is "normal for age" versus concerning is a common theme.

Safety in the clinic involves preventing falls from exam tables, keeping small objects and sharp tools out of reach, and supervising children closely—especially if caregivers are distracted. You may need to use side rails, never leave a small child unattended on a high surface, and ensure that siblings are also safe. The exam favors answers where the CMA takes proactive steps to protect children from injury rather than assuming parents will handle everything.

9.4 Pediatric Immunizations and Well-Child Visits

WELL-CHILD VISITS ARE a cornerstone of pediatric care, often including growth assessment, developmental screening, and immunizations. CMAs are frequently involved in preparing vaccines, assisting with administration, and providing education. The exam expects familiarity with the general purpose and flow of these visits, not memorization of every schedule detail.

- Supporting immunization administration in children
- Assisting with well-child assessments and screenings

Supporting immunizations includes verifying vaccine orders, checking allergies and prior reactions, choosing correct sites and needle sizes by age (per policy), and assisting in safe restraint only when necessary. You should help comfort the child before and after the injection, perhaps by distraction, reassuring words, or involving the caregiver in soothing. Accurate documentation of vaccine name, lot number, manufacturer, site, and route is essential. Exam questions often test whether you screen appropriately and never give vaccines when clear contraindications appear in the history without provider review.

Well-child assessments may involve measuring weight, length/height, head circumference, and sometimes developmental screenings such as questionnaires about milestones. You might ask caregivers about feeding, sleep, behavior, and school performance, depending on the child's age. Your role includes recording information accurately and reporting concerns like developmental delays, failure to thrive, or behavioral red flags. On the exam, correct answers show the CMA gathering structured information and escalating concerns rather than dismissing them.

9.5 Recognizing and Responding to Possible Child Abuse or Neglect

CMAS ARE IN A POSITION to notice signs that might suggest child abuse or neglect. You are not expected to investigate or prove abuse, but you must recognize suspicious patterns and follow reporting laws and policies. The exam uses these scenarios to test ethics, safety, and professional responsibility.

- Physical and behavioral signs that may raise concern
- Mandatory reporting and CMA responsibilities

Physical signs that may raise concern include unexplained bruises, burns, or injuries in unusual locations or patterns, multiple injuries at different stages of healing, or poor hygiene and malnutrition. Behavioral signs can include extreme fearfulness, withdrawal, aggression, or reluctance to be alone with a particular adult. While each sign alone may not prove abuse, patterns combined with an inconsistent or evasive explanation are worrisome. Exam questions often present subtle clinical clues and ask what the CMA should do next.

Mandatory reporting laws usually require healthcare professionals—and often all staff in a clinical setting—to report suspected abuse to appropriate authorities. The CMA's role is to document observations objectively (what was seen and heard) and promptly notify the provider or designated person according to policy so a report can be made. You should not confront the suspected abuser in a way that escalates risk. On the exam, ignoring strong signs of abuse or trying to "handle it yourself" is almost always the wrong choice.

9.6 Geriatric Patients: Physiologic Changes and Assessment

OLDER ADULTS OFTEN experience normal age-related changes in vision, hearing, balance, mobility, and organ function. These changes can affect how they present symptoms and how you assess them. The CMA must differentiate between expected changes and signs that might indicate disease.

- Common age-related changes affecting assessment
- Adapting assessment techniques for older adults

Common age-related changes can include decreased visual acuity, reduced hearing (especially high-frequency sounds), slower reflexes, and changes in blood pressure regulation. Skin becomes more fragile, and thermoregulation may be less reliable, so fevers may be blunted or subtle. Cognitive changes range from normal forgetfulness to more serious impairment. On exam questions, you may need to recognize that "normal for age" does not mean ignoring new or sudden changes, such as acute confusion.

Adapting assessment for older adults might include speaking clearly and facing the patient so they can read lips, allowing extra time for responses, and minimizing background noise. Gentle handling is important to avoid bruising fragile skin or causing discomfort with positioning. You may need to assist with getting on and off exam tables and consider orthostatic vital sign checks. The exam rewards answers where the CMA is patient, respectful, and physically careful, not rushed or dismissive.

9.7 Geriatric Safety, Polypharmacy, and Functional Status

GERIATRIC SAFETY INVOLVES more than avoiding infections—it includes preventing falls, medication errors, and functional decline. Many older adults take multiple medications (polypharmacy), which can increase risks. The CMA often gathers information that helps the provider evaluate safety and independence.

- Fall risk and functional assessment basics
- Polypharmacy awareness and medication reconciliation support

Fall risk may be increased by muscle weakness, balance issues, poor vision, unsafe home environments, and certain medications. You can ask about recent falls, difficulty walking, or needing help with daily activities like bathing or shopping. Observing how a patient moves from chair to exam table can offer clues about mobility. Exam questions often ask what the CMA should note or report when an older adult appears unsteady or has a history of falls.

Polypharmacy occurs when a patient takes many medications, which can interact or cause side effects like dizziness, confusion, or low blood pressure. Medication reconciliation—reviewing all current prescriptions, OTC drugs, supplements, and herbal remedies—helps ensure the list is accurate. The CMA may collect this information and enter it into the record for provider review. On the exam, answers that emphasize accurate lists and reporting possible side effects (like falls or confusion) are considered safe and appropriate.

9.8 Obstetric Patients: Prenatal Visits and Assessment

PREGNANT PATIENTS HAVE unique physical and emotional needs and may be seen frequently for prenatal care. The CMA plays a key role in gathering data, offering support, and reinforcing health teaching. The exam tests whether you understand what's typical in prenatal visits versus what's concerning.

- Routine tasks during prenatal visits
- Recognizing warning signs that require provider attention

Routine prenatal tasks may include measuring weight, blood pressure, documenting gestational age, and collecting urine samples (for protein, glucose, etc.). In later pregnancy, fundal height and fetal heart tones may be assessed by the provider with your assistance. You also verify allergies, medications, and any new symptoms since the last visit. Exam questions often show you prenatal vital signs and symptoms and ask what should be reported.

Warning signs in pregnancy can include severe headache, visual changes, sudden swelling of hands or face, abdominal pain, decreased fetal movement, vaginal bleeding, or leaking fluid. While you don't diagnose, you must recognize these as needing immediate provider attention. The exam tends to reward answers where the CMA takes such symptoms seriously, not attributing them automatically to "normal pregnancy discomfort" without escalation.

9.9 Supporting Pregnant Patients: Comfort, Education, and Sensitivity

PREGNANCY CAN BRING joy, anxiety, physical discomfort, and sometimes complications. CMAs support pregnant patients by being sensitive to their physical limitations and emotional needs. The exam uses scenarios to assess whether you provide appropriate support and patient education within scope.

- Physical comfort, positioning, and mobility considerations

- Basic education reinforcement and emotional support

Physical comfort means recognizing that lying flat on the back may become uncomfortable or unsafe in later pregnancy due to vena cava compression, and that prolonged standing may cause dizziness or swelling. You might help the patient change positions slowly, offer support when getting on and off the table, and allow short rest breaks if needed. On test questions, answers that protect maternal safety and comfort—such as avoiding sudden position changes—are usually correct.

Basic education reinforcement includes encouraging prenatal vitamins as ordered, supporting healthy lifestyle choices, and reinforcing provider instructions on nutrition, activity, and warning signs. Emotionally, you should listen to concerns without judgment, acknowledge fears, and encourage questions. While you don't provide detailed counseling on complex issues, you can direct patients to the provider or appropriate resources. The exam favors responses that show empathy, respect, and clear communication rather than dismissing concerns as "normal" without explanation.

9.10 End-of-Life, Family Dynamics, and Respect Across Populations

SPECIAL POPULATIONS often involve sensitive topics like serious illness in children, frailty in older adults, or high-risk pregnancies. Family dynamics and end-of-life discussions may surface during visits. The CMA is not the decision-maker but must show respect and professionalism in these situations.

- Respecting family roles and cultural values
- Supporting communication around serious or end-of-life issues within scope

Respecting family roles means recognizing that some cultures involve extended family or specific decision-makers, while others emphasize individual autonomy. You should ask patients how they prefer information to be shared and who should be involved. Avoiding assumptions and stereotyping is key. On exam questions, the best answers are those that clarify preferences and involve the right people with the patient's permission.

Supporting communication around serious illness or end-of-life issues includes being present, listening, and avoiding giving false reassurance or personal opinions about treatment choices. You can help schedule family meetings, ensure that the provider knows there are concerns, and provide a calm, respectful presence. You must avoid making promises or decisions that are outside your scope. The exam tends to reward answers where the CMA acknowledges difficulty, respects privacy, and directs complex discussions to the provider or appropriate team members.

Practice Questions – Chapter 9 (25 Questions)

THESE QUESTIONS FOCUS on Chapter 9 content: pediatrics, development, growth/vitals, immunizations, possible abuse, geriatrics, safety and polypharmacy, prenatal/obstetric care, support/education, and family/end-of-life dynamics.

1. When communicating with a 4-year-old child, the CMA should:
   A. Use complex medical terminology to build vocabulary
   B. Speak in simple, concrete terms and possibly use demonstrations or toys
   C. Ignore the child and talk only to the parent
   D. Expect the child to understand adult-level explanations

2. A school-age child asks, "Is this shot going to hurt?" The most appropriate CMA response is:
   A. "No, you won't feel anything at all."
   B. "It might sting for a moment, but I'll be quick and you can hold your parent's hand."
   C. "Don't be a baby; it's nothing."
   D. "If you don't cry, you get better care."
3. A toddler is crying and attempts to stand on the exam table alone. The CMA's **best** action is to:
   A. Step back and let them explore
   B. Stay close, ensure side rails are up or hold the child, and never leave them unattended
   C. Leave the room quickly to get the provider
   D. Give them small objects to play with, even if they are choking hazards
4. A pediatric growth chart shows a child's weight dropping from the 60th to the 15th percentile over several months. The CMA should:
   A. Change the numbers to keep them at the 60th percentile
   B. Document and notify the provider of the significant change
   C. Ignore the chart because children grow unpredictably
   D. Reassure parents without telling the provider
5. Which of the following is a **subjective** sign that may suggest possible child abuse?
   A. Multiple bruises in different healing stages
   B. A child stating, "I'm scared to go home."
   C. Clean clothing and good hygiene
   D. Normal growth percentiles
6. When abuse is suspected, the CMA should:
   A. Investigate the situation personally and confront the caregiver aggressively
   B. Document observations objectively and follow mandatory reporting policies
   C. Ignore suspicions unless proof is certain
   D. Discuss the situation only with friends
7. Which is the **best** example of objective documentation related to suspected abuse?
   A. "Child is probably abused."
   B. "Mom looked guilty."
   C. "Child has 3 oval-shaped bruises approximately 2 cm on right upper arm; child stated, 'I fell,' no other explanation given."
   D. "The family seems suspicious."
8. An older adult patient seems hard of hearing. The CMA should:
   A. Shout directly into one ear
   B. Speak clearly, face the patient, and reduce background noise
   C. Talk from behind to avoid embarrassment
   D. Assume they are confused and ignore them
9. A geriatric patient reports recent falls and dizziness when standing. The CMA's **best** response is to:
   A. Assume this is normal aging and ignore it
   B. Document and notify the provider, and consider orthostatic vital signs if ordered
   C. Tell the patient to stop moving so much
   D. Immediately prescribe a cane
10. An older adult takes multiple prescriptions, OTC medications, and herbal supplements. The CMA should:
    A. Only list prescription medications in the chart

B. Conduct medication reconciliation by listing all substances taken and shared with the provider
C. Tell the patient to stop all supplements without asking the provider
D. Assume the pharmacy already knows everything

11. During a prenatal visit, which task is appropriate for the CMA?
A. Diagnosing pregnancy complications
B. Measuring weight and blood pressure and collecting urine as ordered
C. Interpreting fetal heart tones and giving a prognosis
D. Advising the patient to change prescribed medication without provider input

12. A pregnant patient reports severe headache and visual changes. The CMA should:
A. Assume it is normal and offer reassurance only
B. Provide over-the-counter medication without provider approval
C. Recognize these as warning signs needing prompt provider notification
D. Ignore the symptoms and continue routine care

13. In late pregnancy, lying flat on the back for a long time may cause:
A. Better circulation
B. Vena cava compression leading to dizziness or low blood pressure
C. Stronger bones
D. More effective digestion

14. The CMA helps a late-pregnancy patient off the exam table. The **safest** approach is to:
A. Ask them to sit up quickly and jump down
B. Encourage slow position changes and offer support as they stand
C. Leave the room and let them manage
D. Tell them to lie down again immediately

15. A teenage patient asks to speak privately without their parents in the room about a sensitive health concern. The CMA should:
A. Automatically refuse and insist the parent stays
B. Automatically exclude the parent without explanation
C. Follow clinic policy and applicable laws about adolescent confidentiality, and involve the provider as needed
D. Share everything with the parent without telling the teen

16. During a well-child visit, a parent reports their 2-year-old is not using any words yet. The CMA's best action is to:
A. Ignore it; some children just don't talk
B. Document the concern as possible developmental delay and notify the provider
C. Tell the parent they are overreacting
D. Advise speech therapy immediately without provider review

17. A geriatric patient appears confused today but was alert at the last visit. The CMA should:
A. Assume dementia and do nothing
B. Document the change and notify the provider of new confusion
C. Tell the patient they are just getting old
D. Refuse to take vitals

18. A child presents with multiple bruises in different healing stages and no clear explanation. The CMA should:
A. Accept the vague explanation without question
B. Document findings objectively and report concerns according to policy and law

C. Confront the child aggressively
D. Post about the case on social media

19. A pregnant patient expresses anxiety about labor and says, "I'm scared I won't be able to handle it." The CMA's most appropriate response is:
A. "You're worrying for no reason."
B. "It's understandable to feel scared. Let's talk about your questions, and I can let the provider know you'd like more information about pain options."
C. "You shouldn't think about that."
D. "Just be tough."
20. For older adults at high fall risk, which observation should the CMA be sure to report?
A. Preference for reading books
B. Difficulty stepping up onto the exam table and needing to grab furniture
C. Enjoyment of walking outside
D. Drinking water frequently
21. A parent declines a recommended vaccine for their child. The CMA should:
A. Yell at the parent for endangering the child
B. Respectfully provide accurate information, answer questions, and notify the provider of the refusal
C. Secretly give the vaccine anyway
D. Tell the family they are no longer welcome at the clinic
22. In discussing serious illness or end-of-life issues with a family, the CMA's role typically includes:
A. Making treatment decisions for the family
B. Giving personal opinions about what they should choose
C. Providing a calm, respectful presence, listening, and directing complex decisions to the provider or appropriate team
D. Sharing confidential details with other patients
23. A geriatric patient appears unkempt, with dirty clothing and poor hygiene, and reports difficulty bathing alone. The CMA should:
A. Ignore this because appearance is not medical
B. Document the observation and inform the provider, as it may indicate functional decline or need for support
C. Make jokes about their appearance
D. Tell them to "try harder"
24. A pregnant patient asks if the CMA can interpret her ultrasound results. The CMA should respond by:
A. Giving a full interpretation based on the picture
B. Saying, "The provider will review your ultrasound and explain what it means; I'll make sure they know you have questions."
C. Refusing to talk at all
D. Guessing based on the baby's size on the screen
25. At the end of a difficult visit where a child was diagnosed with a serious condition, the CMA's most appropriate action is to:
A. Insist the family stop crying and leave quickly
B. Offer tissues, speak gently, and ensure they know when and how to reach the provider with further questions, staying within scope
C. Promise the child they will definitely be cured

D. Give detailed treatment advice beyond the provider's instructions

Answer Key – Chapter 9 (with Justifications)

1. **B** – Simple, concrete language and demonstrations help a 4-year-old understand and feel less afraid.
2. **B** – This response is honest, sets realistic expectations, and offers comfort and support.
3. **B** – Young children should never be left unattended on exam tables; maintaining close supervision and safety measures prevents falls.
4. **B** – A significant drop in growth percentile warrants documentation and provider notification for evaluation.
5. **B** – A child saying "I'm scared to go home" is subjective but concerning and should be documented and considered alongside other findings.
6. **B** – CMAs must document observations objectively and follow mandatory reporting policies; they should not investigate on their own or ignore concerns.
7. **C** – This statement describes specific, objective findings and the child's statement without labeling or assumptions.
8. **B** – Speaking clearly, facing the patient, and reducing noise support communication with hearing difficulties without shouting or disrespect.
9. **B** – Falls and orthostatic-like symptoms are not automatically "normal aging" and require documentation and provider attention.
10. **B** – Full medication reconciliation, including prescriptions, OTCs, and supplements, helps the provider evaluate polypharmacy risks.
11. **B** – Measuring weight, BP, and collecting urine are typical CMA tasks at prenatal visits; diagnosis and medication changes are provider roles.
12. **C** – Severe headaches and visual changes in pregnancy can be warning signs and must be reported promptly.
13. **B** – Lying flat in late pregnancy can compress the vena cava, causing dizziness or hypotension.
14. **B** – Older pregnant patients may need slow position changes and physical support to prevent falls and dizziness.
15. **C** – Adolescent confidentiality is guided by law and policy; the CMA should follow these and involve the provider as needed.
16. **B** – Lack of any words at 2 years may indicate developmental delay; documenting and notifying the provider is appropriate.
17. **B** – New confusion is a change from baseline and could indicate acute illness; it must be documented and reported.
18. **B** – Multiple unexplained bruises in different healing stages require objective documentation and reporting under abuse policies.
19. **B** – Acknowledging fear, offering information, and involving the provider is supportive and within scope.
20. **B** – Difficulty climbing onto the table and grabbing furniture suggests fall risk and should be reported to the provider.
21. **B** – Respectful education and provider notification balance patient autonomy with safety; secret administration or hostility is inappropriate.
22. **C** – The CMA supports communication and directs decisions to the provider, maintaining professionalism and patient/family respect.
23. **B** – Poor hygiene and difficulty bathing may reflect functional decline or social issues; documenting and notifying the provider is important.

24. **B** – Ultrasound interpretation is the provider's role; the CMA should ensure the provider knows the patient has questions.
25. **B** – Offering simple comfort, clear follow-up information, and staying within scope is appropriate after a difficult diagnosis.

Chapter 10

Anatomy & Physiology Essentials for the CMA

You don't need to be a physician-level anatomy expert to pass the CMA exam, but you *do* need a solid working map of the human body. Knowing how major systems are structured and how they function helps you understand vital signs, exam findings, and medical terminology. This chapter gives you a high-yield overview of key anatomy and physiology concepts that show up frequently in CMA questions.

10.1 Levels of Organization: From Cells to Organ Systems

THE BODY IS ORGANIZED in layers, starting from tiny units and building up to entire organ systems. Understanding these levels gives you a framework to place signs, symptoms, and treatments into context. The exam often uses terminology linked to these levels.

- Basic levels of organization in the human body
- The role of cells as functional units

The basic levels of organization include cells, tissues, organs, organ systems, and the whole organism. Cells combine to form tissues, tissues form organs like the heart or lungs, and organs work together in systems like the cardiovascular or respiratory systems. Each level depends on the proper function of the ones below it, so problems at the cellular level can eventually show up as disease at the system level. On the exam, answers that connect symptoms to the correct body system or structure often rely on this layered understanding.

Cells are the smallest units of life that can perform all necessary functions, such as obtaining energy, eliminating waste, and reproducing. Different cell types have specialized structures—like muscle cells that contract or nerve cells that transmit signals. When too many cells become damaged or die, tissues and organs cannot function normally. The CMA exam expects you to recognize that many diseases start with cellular injury or dysfunction, even if you don't go into microscopic detail.

10.2 Tissues, Membranes, and Basic Body Planes

TISSUES ARE GROUPS of similar cells working together, and membranes line and protect structures in the body. Body planes and directional terms help describe locations and movements precisely. The exam uses this language regularly when describing injuries, procedures, and anatomy.

- Four basic tissue types and common examples
- Body planes and directional terms used in healthcare

The four main tissue types are epithelial, connective, muscle, and nervous tissue. Epithelial tissue lines surfaces and forms glands, such as skin and the lining of the GI tract. Connective tissue supports and binds, including bone, blood, and cartilage. Muscle tissue contracts to produce movement, and nervous tissue conducts impulses for communication. On exam questions, recognizing which tissue is involved can help you understand conditions like skin cancers (epithelial) or muscle injuries.

Body planes—such as sagittal (left/right), frontal or coronal (front/back), and transverse or horizontal (top/bottom)—are imaginary lines used to slice the body in descriptive ways. Directional terms like anterior/posterior, superior/inferior, medial/lateral, and proximal/distal describe locations relative to other structures. For example, the wrist is distal to the elbow, and the sternum is anterior to the spine. The CMA exam uses these terms in charting scenarios and procedure descriptions, so knowing them lets you decode anatomical directions quickly.

10.3 Homeostasis and Body Regulation

HOMEOSTASIS IS THE body's way of keeping internal conditions within a narrow, healthy range. Even when the outside world changes, your internal environment (like temperature and fluid balance) stays relatively stable. The CMA exam often tests whether you understand this idea when interpreting vital signs and lab values.

- The concept of homeostasis and feedback mechanisms
- Examples of homeostatic balance in daily practice

Homeostasis involves continuous monitoring and adjustment by body systems using feedback loops, often negative feedback. For example, when body temperature rises, mechanisms like sweating and vasodilation help cool it down; when it falls, shivering and vasoconstriction help warm it up. Endocrine and nervous systems play major roles in detecting changes and coordinating responses. On the exam, understanding homeostasis helps explain why extreme temperatures, dehydration, or blood sugar imbalances are dangerous.

Everyday examples include maintaining blood pressure, blood glucose, and fluid and electrolyte levels. If blood pressure drops, the heart may beat faster and vessels constrict to restore adequate circulation. If blood glucose rises after a meal, hormones like insulin help move glucose into cells and lower blood sugar. When homeostasis fails, you see conditions like shock, uncontrolled diabetes, or heat stroke. The CMA must recognize when vital signs suggest the body is struggling to maintain balance and report it promptly.

10.4 Cardiovascular System: Heart and Blood Vessels

THE CARDIOVASCULAR system pumps blood throughout the body, delivering oxygen and nutrients and removing waste. It's central to vital signs, emergencies, and many chronic diseases. The CMA exam frequently includes questions about heart function, blood pressure, and circulation.

- Structure and basic function of the heart
- Blood vessels and circulation pathways

The heart has four chambers—two atria and two ventricles—and valves that keep blood flowing in the right direction. The right side pumps deoxygenated blood to the lungs (pulmonary circulation), while the left side pumps oxygenated blood to the body (systemic circulation). Electrical activity in the heart coordinates contractions, which is what ECGs measure. On the exam, knowing which side pumps where and understanding terms like "ventricle" or "atrium" helps when interpreting basic cardiovascular questions.

Blood vessels include arteries (carrying blood away from the heart), veins (returning blood to the heart), and capillaries (where exchanges of gases and nutrients occur). Blood pressure reflects the force of blood against artery walls and is affected by cardiac output and vessel resistance. Poor circulation can lead to symptoms like cool extremities, edema, or chest pain. The CMA frequently measures blood pressure and pulse, and the exam expects you to associate extremely abnormal values with potential cardiovascular problems.

10.5 Respiratory System: Gas Exchange and Breathing

THE RESPIRATORY SYSTEM brings oxygen into the body and removes carbon dioxide. It closely interacts with the cardiovascular system to maintain adequate oxygen delivery to tissues. The exam often tests your understanding of basic respiratory anatomy and what abnormal breathing might mean.

- Major respiratory structures and airflow path
- Gas exchange and factors affecting breathing

Air enters through the nose or mouth, passes through the pharynx, larynx, trachea, and bronchi, and then into progressively smaller bronchioles ending in alveoli. The lungs are housed in the thoracic cavity and surrounded by pleural membranes. The diaphragm and intercostal muscles drive breathing by changing chest volume and pressure. On exam questions, recognizing terms like trachea, bronchi, or alveoli helps you place where conditions like bronchitis or pneumonia occur.

Gas exchange occurs in the alveoli, tiny air sacs where oxygen moves into the blood and carbon dioxide moves out. Effective ventilation depends on open airways, functioning lung tissue, and proper chest wall movement. Conditions like asthma, COPD, or pneumonia can impair gas exchange and cause shortness of breath, wheezing, or low oxygen levels. The CMA must recognize signs of respiratory distress such as rapid breathing, use of accessory muscles, or cyanosis and report them as potential emergencies.

10.6 Nervous System: Control and Communication

THE NERVOUS SYSTEM acts as the body's rapid communication network, coordinating activities and responses. It includes the central nervous system (CNS) and peripheral nervous system (PNS). The exam uses neurological concepts to frame questions about mental status, reflexes, and certain emergencies like stroke.

- Central and peripheral nervous system basics
- Sensory, motor, and autonomic functions

The CNS consists of the brain and spinal cord, which process information and send commands. The PNS includes all the nerves that branch out to the rest of the body. Some nerves carry sensory information inward, while others carry motor commands outward. Damage to certain areas can affect movement, sensation, speech, or cognition. On the CMA exam, recognizing changes like sudden weakness on one side or slurred speech as possible neurological issues is important.

Sensory nerves carry signals like pain, temperature, and touch to the CNS, while motor nerves send signals to muscles to produce movement. The autonomic nervous system (ANS) regulates involuntary functions such as heart rate, digestion, and blood vessel tone; it has sympathetic ("fight or flight") and parasympathetic ("rest and digest") divisions. For example, sympathetic activation increases heart rate and dilates pupils, while parasympathetic activity slows the heart and promotes digestion. The exam may ask about these responses in stress, shock, or medication effects.

10.7 Endocrine System: Hormones and Metabolism

THE ENDOCRINE SYSTEM uses hormones to regulate processes like growth, metabolism, and reproduction. Hormones travel through the blood to target organs and adjust their activity. The CMA exam often includes basic questions about diabetes, thyroid disorders, and other endocrine conditions.

- Major endocrine glands and their general roles
- Hormone regulation and common clinical examples

Major endocrine glands include the pituitary, thyroid, parathyroids, adrenals, pancreas (endocrine portion), and gonads (ovaries and testes). The pituitary is often called the "master gland" because it releases hormones that influence other glands. The thyroid regulates metabolism and energy use, while the adrenals help manage stress responses and fluid balance. On the exam, you may be asked to connect symptoms like weight changes, fatigue, or intolerance to heat or cold to thyroid function conceptually.

Hormone regulation often uses feedback loops, where levels in the blood signal glands to increase or decrease secretion. For example, when blood glucose rises, the pancreas releases insulin to help cells absorb glucose, lowering blood sugar. Diabetes mellitus involves problems with insulin production or response, leading to high blood sugar and complications. The CMA must recognize signs of high or low blood glucose, such as excessive thirst, frequent urination, confusion, or shakiness, and respond appropriately by reporting them.

10.8 Digestive System: From Ingestion to Elimination

THE DIGESTIVE (GASTROINTESTINAL) system breaks down food, absorbs nutrients, and eliminates waste. Many common complaints in the clinic—like abdominal pain, nausea, or constipation—relate to this system. The exam expects you to know the basic anatomy and general function of key organs.

- Major digestive organs and their functions
- Absorption, elimination, and common GI symptoms

The digestive tract runs from the mouth to the anus and includes the esophagus, stomach, small intestine, and large intestine. Accessory organs like the liver, gallbladder, and pancreas produce substances that aid digestion, such as bile and digestive enzymes. The stomach mainly performs mechanical mixing and initial chemical breakdown, while most nutrient absorption occurs in the small intestine. On exam questions, matching symptoms to likely locations—like upper abdominal pain with stomach issues or right-upper-quadrant pain with gallbladder—can be helpful.

The large intestine absorbs water and forms stool for elimination. When transit is too fast, diarrhea can result; when it's too slow, constipation may occur. Disorders like GERD, ulcers, irritable bowel syndrome, or inflammatory bowel disease affect specific parts of the GI tract and produce characteristic symptoms such as heartburn, cramping, or blood in stool. The CMA is often involved in stool sample handling, patient education on diet, and recognizing when GI symptoms might need urgent attention, such as severe pain or black, tarry stools.

10.9 Urinary System and Fluid Balance

THE URINARY SYSTEM filters blood, removes waste, and helps regulate fluid and electrolyte balance. It also plays a role in blood pressure control. The CMA exam frequently touches on urinary symptoms, kidney function basics, and urine testing.

- Kidneys, ureters, bladder, and urethra functions
- Fluid balance, urine characteristics, and common urinary symptoms

The kidneys filter the blood to remove waste products and excess fluid, producing urine. Urine then travels down the ureters to the bladder, where it is stored until voiding through the urethra. Damage to the kidneys can lead to waste buildup and electrolyte imbalances, affecting many systems. On exam questions, you'll often see urinary complaints (painful urination, frequency, blood in urine) that point to issues in this system.

Fluid balance requires a balance between intake (drinking, food, IV fluids) and output (urine, sweat, breathing). The kidneys adjust urine concentration to conserve or excrete water and electrolytes like sodium and potassium. Urine characteristics—such as color, clarity, odor, and presence of blood or protein—can offer clues about health. The CMA frequently collects urine samples and must recognize when symptoms like burning, urgency, flank pain, or little urine output might indicate infection or other kidney/urinary problems that need provider attention.

10.10 Integumentary and Musculoskeletal Systems

THE INTEGUMENTARY SYSTEM (skin, hair, nails) protects the body, while the musculoskeletal system supports movement and posture. Many routine assessments involve skin inspection and musculoskeletal checks. The CMA exam expects basic knowledge of these systems and how problems show up in practice.

- Skin structure, functions, and common issues
- Bones, muscles, joints, and movement basics

Skin has three main layers: epidermis (outer), dermis (middle), and subcutaneous tissue (deep). It acts as a barrier, helps regulate temperature, and provides sensory information. Common issues include rashes, infections, pressure injuries, and wounds. Changes in skin color (pallor, cyanosis, jaundice), temperature, or turgor can signal systemic problems like poor circulation, oxygenation issues, or dehydration. On the exam, recognizing these signs can guide you to select safe actions such as reporting findings promptly.

The musculoskeletal system includes bones that provide structure, muscles that produce movement, and joints where bones meet and allow motion. Ligaments connect bone to bone, and tendons connect muscle to bone. Injuries such as sprains, strains, fractures, and arthritis affect these structures and can limit mobility and cause pain. The CMA may assist with applying splints, supports, or teaching about activity modification. Exam questions often ask you to match symptoms like joint swelling, limited range of motion, or deformity to musculoskeletal concerns that require provider evaluation.

Practice Questions – Chapter 10 (25 Questions)

THESE QUESTIONS FOCUS on Chapter 10 content: levels of organization, tissues/planes, homeostasis, cardiovascular, respiratory, nervous, endocrine, digestive, urinary, integumentary, and musculoskeletal basics.

1. Which of the following lists the levels of organization from **smallest to largest**?
   A. Organ → cell → tissue → system
   B. Cell → tissue → organ → organ system → organism
   C. Tissue → cell → organ → organism → system
   D. Cell → organ → tissue → system → organism
2. A group of similar cells working together to perform a specific function is called a:
   A. System
   B. Tissue
   C. Organ
   D. Membrane
3. Which type of tissue primarily lines body surfaces and forms glands?
   A. Muscle tissue
   B. Nervous tissue
   C. Epithelial tissue
   D. Connective tissue
4. The plane that divides the body into left and right portions is called the:
   A. Coronal (frontal) plane
   B. Transverse plane
   C. Sagittal plane
   D. Horizontal plane
5. The term **proximal** means:
   A. Toward the head
   B. Toward the midline
   C. Closer to the point of attachment
   D. Farther away from the surface
6. Homeostasis is best described as:
   A. The body's inability to change
   B. The body's attempt to maintain a stable internal environment
   C. The process of breaking down nutrients
   D. The formation of blood cells
7. Which of the following is an example of homeostatic control?
   A. Hair growing longer over time
   B. Sweating when body temperature rises
   C. Nails breaking
   D. Tattoos on skin
8. The right side of the heart primarily pumps blood to the:
   A. Brain
   B. Lungs
   C. Liver
   D. Kidneys
9. Arteries generally:
   A. Carry blood toward the heart
   B. Carry blood away from the heart
   C. Only carry deoxygenated blood

D. Only carry oxygenated blood

10. Gas exchange between air and blood primarily occurs in the:
    A. Trachea
    B. Bronchi
    C. Alveoli
    D. Pleura
11. Which sign would most strongly suggest **respiratory distress** in a patient?
    A. Calm speech in full sentences
    B. Slow, regular breathing at rest
    C. Use of neck muscles to breathe and inability to speak full sentences
    D. Mild yawning
12. The central nervous system consists of the:
    A. Brain and spinal cord
    B. Brain and cranial nerves
    C. Spinal cord and peripheral nerves
    D. Heart and blood vessels
13. The "fight or flight" response is primarily controlled by the:
    A. Parasympathetic nervous system
    B. Sympathetic nervous system
    C. Somatic nervous system
    D. Digestive system
14. The thyroid gland mainly helps regulate:
    A. Blood clotting
    B. Metabolism and energy use
    C. Urine production
    D. Lung capacity
15. A patient with diabetes mellitus has a problem related to which hormone system?
    A. Insulin regulation and blood glucose control
    B. Thyroid hormone and metabolism
    C. Estrogen production
    D. Calcium regulation only
16. Most nutrient absorption takes place in the:
    A. Stomach
    B. Small intestine
    C. Large intestine
    D. Esophagus
17. Which accessory organ produces bile to help digest fats?
    A. Pancreas
    B. Liver
    C. Spleen
    D. Kidney
18. The main function of the kidneys is to:
    A. Pump blood throughout the body
    B. Produce digestive enzymes

C. Filter blood, remove waste, and help regulate fluid balance
D. Control body temperature

19. A patient reports burning with urination and increased frequency. These symptoms most likely involve which system?
A. Respiratory system
B. Musculoskeletal system
C. Urinary system
D. Nervous system
20. Which skin finding would be most concerning and should be reported promptly?
A. Warm, pink skin after exercise
B. Sudden bluish coloration of lips and fingernails
C. Mild tanning after vacation
D. Temporary redness from tight clothing
21. The outermost layer of the skin is the:
A. Dermis
B. Epidermis
C. Subcutaneous tissue
D. Fascia
22. A fracture is best defined as a:
A. Torn tendon
B. Sprained ligament
C. Break or crack in a bone
D. Bruise in a muscle
23. Ligaments connect:
A. Muscle to bone
B. Bone to bone
C. Muscle to muscle
D. Skin to muscle
24. A patient presents with swollen, painful knee joints and limited movement. These symptoms most directly involve the:
A. Nervous system
B. Musculoskeletal system (joints)
C. Respiratory system
D. Integumentary system
25. A CMA notices that a patient's blood pressure is dropping and pulse is rising, and the patient feels dizzy and cold. These changes suggest the body may be:
A. In perfect homeostasis
B. Struggling to maintain circulation, possibly indicating shock
C. Experiencing normal rest
D. Adjusting to mild exercise only

Answer Key – Chapter 10 (with Justifications)

1. **B** – The correct order from smallest to largest is cell → tissue → organ → organ system → organism.

2. **B** – Tissues are groups of similar cells that work together to perform specific functions.
3. **C** – Epithelial tissue lines surfaces and forms glands, including skin and mucous membranes.
4. **C** – The sagittal plane divides the body into left and right portions.
5. **C** – Proximal means closer to the point of attachment or to the trunk of the body.
6. **B** – Homeostasis is the body's effort to maintain a stable internal environment despite external changes.
7. **B** – Sweating to cool the body when temperature rises is a classic example of homeostatic control.
8. **B** – The right side of the heart pumps deoxygenated blood to the lungs for oxygenation.
9. **B** – Arteries, by definition, carry blood away from the heart (whether oxygenated or not).
10. **C** – Gas exchange takes place in the alveoli, where oxygen enters blood and carbon dioxide leaves.
11. **C** – Use of accessory muscles and inability to speak full sentences suggest significant respiratory distress.
12. **A** – The central nervous system includes the brain and spinal cord.
13. **B** – The sympathetic nervous system controls "fight or flight" responses, increasing heart rate and alertness.
14. **B** – The thyroid gland primarily regulates metabolism and energy use.
15. **A** – Diabetes mellitus involves problems with insulin production or action, affecting blood glucose regulation.
16. **B** – Most nutrient absorption occurs in the small intestine.
17. **B** – The liver produces bile, which helps emulsify fats for digestion.
18. **C** – Kidneys filter blood, remove waste as urine, and help regulate fluid and electrolyte balance.
19. **C** – Burning and frequency with urination point to issues in the urinary system, such as possible infection.
20. **B** – Sudden cyanosis (bluish lips/nails) may indicate serious oxygenation or circulation problems and must be reported urgently.
21. **B** – The epidermis is the outermost layer of the skin.
22. **C** – A fracture is a break or crack in a bone.
23. **B** – Ligaments connect bone to bone, stabilizing joints.
24. **B** – Swollen, painful joints with limited movement primarily involve the musculoskeletal system, specifically the joints.
25. **B** – Falling blood pressure with rising pulse and symptoms like dizziness and feeling cold suggest compromised circulation and possible shock, not stable homeostasis.

Chapter 11

Medical Terminology and Abbreviations

Medical terminology is like a shared language for healthcare teams. Once you understand the building blocks—prefixes, roots, and suffixes—you can often "decode" unfamiliar words on the CMA exam and in real practice. This chapter focuses on high-yield word parts, common terms, and abbreviations, especially those that impact safety and documentation.

11.1 Word Parts: Prefixes, Roots, and Suffixes

MOST MEDICAL TERMS are built from a combination of prefixes, word roots, and suffixes. Learning these parts helps you guess the meaning of new terms even if you've never seen them before. The CMA exam often expects you to interpret or match terms to their meanings.

- Prefixes that modify meaning (location, time, amount)
- Roots and suffixes that describe body parts and conditions

Prefixes appear at the beginning of words and can describe location ("sub-" = under, "peri-" = around), time ("pre-" = before, "post-" = after), or amount ("hyper-" = excessive, "hypo-" = below/low). For example, "subcutaneous" means under the skin, and "hyperglycemia" means high blood sugar. Recognizing these patterns lets you quickly interpret terms in exam questions and clinical notes without memorizing every single word.

Roots usually refer to body parts or systems, like "cardi/o" (heart), "gastr/o" (stomach), or "neur/o" (nerve). Suffixes often indicate a condition ("-itis" = inflammation, "-oma" = tumor), procedure ("-ectomy" = removal, "-scopy" = visual exam), or specialist ("-logist" = specialist in). When you combine these, "carditis" means inflammation of the heart, and "gastroscopy" means visual examination of the stomach. On the exam, you'll often see questions that test whether you can break a term into its parts and pick the correct definition.

11.2 Common Roots and Terms by Body System

GROUPING ROOTS BY BODY system makes terminology easier to learn and remember. When you know that certain roots belong to cardiology or dermatology, you can spot patterns quickly. The CMA exam often references these roots in questions about diagnosis, procedures, and documentation.

- Cardiovascular, respiratory, and GI system roots
- Musculoskeletal, nervous, and integumentary system roots

Cardiovascular terms often involve roots like "cardi/o" (heart), "angi/o" or "vas/o" (vessel), and "hem/o" or "hemat/o" (blood). Respiratory roots include "pulmon/o" or "pneum/o" (lung), "trache/o" (trachea), and "bronch/o" (bronchus). GI roots include "gastr/o" (stomach), "enter/o" (intestine), "hepat/o" (liver), and "chol/e" (bile). When the exam mentions "hepatitis," for example, knowing "hepat/o" = liver and "-itis" = inflammation tells you this is liver inflammation.

Musculoskeletal terms use roots like "oste/o" (bone), "my/o" (muscle), "arthr/o" (joint), and "tendin/o" (tendon). Nervous system roots include "neur/o" (nerve), "encephal/o" (brain), and "myel/o" (spinal cord or bone marrow, depending on context). Integumentary terms use "derm/o" or "dermat/o" (skin), "trich/o" (hair), and "onych/o" (nail). When you see "osteoporosis," "arthritis," or "dermatitis" on the exam, recognizing the roots and suffixes helps you understand what system and condition are being described.

11.3 Directional, Positional, and Movement Terms

DIRECTIONAL AND POSITIONAL terms are used constantly in charting, imaging, and procedure descriptions. Movement terms describe how joints move and are common in musculoskeletal documentation. The CMA exam often includes these to test your ability to understand written orders or notes.

- Directional and positional terms (anterior, posterior, proximal, distal, etc.)
- Movement terms (flexion, extension, abduction, adduction, etc.)

Directional terms include "anterior" (front) and "posterior" (back), "medial" (toward midline) and "lateral" (away from midline), and "superior" (above) and "inferior" (below). "Proximal" means closer to the point of attachment, while "distal" means farther away. For example, the knee is proximal to the ankle, and the sternum is anterior to the heart. On the exam, if a question describes pain on the "lateral aspect of the right ankle," you should know this refers to the outer side.

Movement terms describe how body parts move at joints. "Flexion" bends a joint, decreasing the angle, while "extension" straightens it. "Abduction" moves a limb away from the midline, and "adduction" brings it back toward the midline. "Rotation" and "circumduction" involve turning or circular movements. The CMA may see these terms in physical therapy orders or exam notes, and the test may ask you to match them to plain-language descriptions like "bending the elbow" or "lifting the arm out to the side."

11.4 Pathology Suffixes: Diseases, Conditions, and Symptoms

MANY MEDICAL TERMS describe diseases, conditions, or symptoms using specific suffixes. Recognizing these endings helps you understand what type of problem is being described. The CMA exam frequently uses these in questions about diagnosis, lab results, and chart entries.

- Suffixes indicating conditions and diseases
- Suffixes related to symptoms or abnormal findings

Common condition-related suffixes include "-itis" (inflammation), "-osis" (abnormal condition), "-oma" (tumor), and "-pathy" (disease). For example, "arthritis" is joint inflammation, "dermatosis" is a skin condition, and "neuropathy" is a nerve disease. "Carcinoma" and "sarcoma" often indicate malignant tumors arising from different tissue types. When you see a term ending in "-itis" on the exam, you can quickly assume inflammation is involved, even before you recall details.

Symptom-related suffixes include "-algia" (pain), "-dynia" (pain), "-rrhea" (flow/discharge), "-emia" (blood condition), and "-plegia" (paralysis). "Myalgia" is muscle pain, "diarrhea" is excessive flow of loose stool, and "anemia" refers to low red blood cell or hemoglobin levels. "Hemiplegia" means paralysis on one side of the body. Recognizing these suffixes helps you interpret complaints or diagnoses like "neuralgia" (nerve pain) or "leukemia" (blood cancer involving white cells) on exam questions and in documentation.

11.5 Procedure and Treatment Suffixes

MANY PROCEDURES AND treatments share common suffixes that describe what is being done. Understanding these helps you interpret orders and know what to expect during a procedure. The CMA exam frequently uses procedure terms in clinical scenarios.

- Surgical procedure suffixes (-ectomy, -otomy, -plasty, etc.)
- Diagnostic and treatment-related suffixes (-scopy, -gram, -therapy, etc.)

Surgical suffixes include "-ectomy" (removal/excision), "-otomy" (cutting into), "-ostomy" (creating an opening), and "-plasty" (surgical repair). For example, "appendectomy" is removal of the appendix, "tracheostomy" is creating an opening in the trachea, and "rhinoplasty" is surgical reshaping of the nose. On the exam, recognizing these endings helps you quickly identify whether a term refers to removing something, repairing it, or creating an opening.

Diagnostic and treatment-related suffixes include "-scopy" (visual examination with a scope), "-gram" (record or image), "-graphy" (process of recording), and "-therapy" (treatment). "Endoscopy" is internal visual examination, "mammogram" is an x-ray image of the breast, and "chemotherapy" refers to chemical treatment, usually for cancer. The CMA will often assist with or prepare for procedures whose names include these suffixes, and the exam expects you to match terms like "colonoscopy" or "electrocardiogram" with the correct basic description.

11.6 Number, Size, and Color Prefixes

A SURPRISING NUMBER of medical terms use prefixes related to number, size, and color. These clues can quickly tell you how many structures are involved, how big something is, or what it looks like. The CMA exam may slip these terms into questions about conditions or test results.

- Number and size prefixes (mono-, bi-, poly-, micro-, macro-, etc.)
- Color-related prefixes and what they usually indicate

Number prefixes include "mono-" (one), "bi-" (two), "tri-" (three), and "poly-" (many). For example, "monocyte" is a type of white blood cell with one nucleus, "bicuspid" describes a two-pointed structure, and "polyuria" means excessive urination. Size prefixes include "micro-" (small) and "macro-" (large), such as "microorganism" (tiny organism) or "macrocyte" (large cell). On the exam, recognizing "poly-" vs. "oligo-" (few) can change the meaning of a diagnosis or symptom.

Color prefixes include "erythr/o" (red), "leuk/o" (white), "cyan/o" (blue), "melan/o" (black), and "xanth/o" (yellow). "Cyanosis" literally refers to bluish discoloration, often from low oxygen; "erythema" involves redness, usually from increased blood flow. "Melanoma" is a malignant tumor of pigment-producing cells, and "jaundice" (often associated with yellowing) connects to "xanth-" roots in some terms. The exam may ask you to interpret skin or lab findings based on these color cues, especially cyanosis and pallor.

11.7 Common General Medical Terms and Abbreviations

SOME MEDICAL TERMS and abbreviations show up constantly in charts and exam questions. These might describe timing, routes, or general clinical concepts. The CMA exam expects you to recognize many of these without confusion.

- General terms used in orders and documentation (PRN, STAT, NPO, etc.)
- Common route and timing abbreviations (PO, IM, BID, QID, etc.)

General abbreviations include "PRN" (as needed), "STAT" (immediately), and "NPO" (nothing by mouth). "Dx" stands for diagnosis, "Tx" for treatment, and "Hx" for history. "SOB" stands for shortness of breath, though you should be careful using it in front of patients due to misunderstandings. On the exam, recognizing that "NPO after midnight" means the patient must not eat or drink after midnight is essential for safe pre-procedure preparation.

Route abbreviations include "PO" (by mouth), "IM" (intramuscular), "IV" (intravenous), "SubQ" or "SC" (subcutaneous), and "PR" (per rectum). Timing abbreviations include "QD" or "daily" (once a day), "BID" (twice a day), "TID" (three times a day), "QID" (four times a day), and "Q4H" (every four hours). Some older abbreviations like "QOD" (every other day) may be discouraged due to safety concerns. On the CMA exam, matching the correct route and frequency to a safe administration plan is often key to getting the question right.

11.8 High-Risk Abbreviations and Safety

NOT ALL ABBREVIATIONS are safe; some are prone to misinterpretation and are discouraged or banned by many facilities. Using or misreading these can lead to medication errors. The CMA exam emphasizes safety and may ask which abbreviation is safest to use or how to clarify an unclear order.

- Examples of unsafe or confusing abbreviations
- Safer alternatives and the importance of clarity

High-risk abbreviations can include "U" for units (mistaken for 0), "IU" (unit confusion), "QD/QOD" (mix-ups with each other), and trailing zeroes like "1.0 mg" (which can be misread as "10 mg"). Some letter combinations, like "MS" or "$MgSO_4$," can be confused with different drugs or doses. Many institutions maintain a "do-not-use" list that staff must follow. On the exam, if you see an option using one of these risky abbreviations, it is often not the best choice.

Safer alternatives include writing "units" instead of "U," "daily" instead of "QD," and avoiding leading/trailing zeroes (using "1 mg," not "1.0 mg"). When any abbreviation is unclear, the safest response is to clarify with the provider rather than guessing. The CMA must treat legibility and clarity as safety priorities, especially in medication orders and documentation. Exam questions often reward answers that replace ambiguous shorthand with clear, fully written terms.

11.9 EHR, Documentation, and Common Charting Shorthand

ELECTRONIC HEALTH RECORDS (EHRs) often include built-in terminology, templates, and abbreviations. While some shorthand is standard, documentation must still be clear and professional. The CMA exam tests how you interpret and use common charting terms appropriately.

- Common charting phrases and symbols (c/o, WNL, ↑, ↓, etc.)
- Using terminology in objective, professional documentation

Common chart abbreviations in charting may include "c/o" (complains of), "WNL" (within normal limits), "Hx" (history), "Pt" (patient), and arrows like "↑" for increased or "↓" for decreased. You might see "BP ↑ from baseline" or "Pt c/o nausea." While these abbreviations are widely used, you should follow facility policy on what is acceptable and avoid creating your own unofficial shorthand. On the exam, being able to translate "Pt c/o SOB x 2 days" into plain language (patient reports shortness of breath for two days) is important.

Objective, professional documentation uses medical terminology accurately but avoids judgmental language. Instead of writing "patient being difficult," you might write "patient refused blood draw after explanation; provider notified." Terms like "alert and oriented x3" describe mental status, while "PRN" or "Stat" may appear in orders. The CMA exam often tests whether your chart entries are clear, specific, and free of slang or personal opinions while correctly using standard terms.

11.10 Pronunciation, Patient-Friendly Language, and Communication

KNOWING MEDICAL TERMINOLOGY is not just about impressing colleagues; it's also about translating complex terms into language patients can understand. The CMA often acts as a bridge between provider language and patient comprehension. The exam may include scenarios where you must choose the best way to explain medical terms to patients.

- Translating medical terms into plain language for patients
- Using terminology correctly when communicating with the healthcare team

Translating terms means turning "hypertension" into "high blood pressure," "myocardial infarction" into "heart attack," or "benign tumor" into "a non-cancerous growth." You should avoid overwhelming patients with jargon and instead check for understanding using simple explanations and teach-back. This helps patients follow instructions and feel more in control of their health. The exam tends to favor responses that simplify language for patients while remaining accurate.

When communicating with providers and other staff, you should use medical terminology correctly and concisely. Misusing terms can cause confusion—for example, confusing "hypoglycemia" (low blood sugar) with "hyperglycemia" (high blood sugar). Pronunciation doesn't need to be perfect, but the meaning must be clear and correct. On the CMA exam, answers that demonstrate both accurate use of terms with the team and patient-friendly translations for teaching usually reflect safe, effective communication.

Practice Questions – Chapter 11 (25 Questions)

THESE QUESTIONS FOCUS on word parts, system roots, directional terms, pathology/procedure suffixes, numbers/colors, common abbreviations, high-risk abbreviations, documentation shorthand, and patient-friendly translations.

1. In the term **"cardiomegaly,"** the suffix **-megaly** means:
   A. Inflammation
   B. Enlargement
   C. Pain
   D. Tumor
2. The prefix **"hypo-"** in the term "hypoglycemia" means:
   A. Excessive
   B. Normal
   C. Below/low

D. Fast

3. The root **"hepat/o"** refers to the:
   A. Heart
   B. Stomach
   C. Kidney
   D. Liver
4. Which term means **inflammation of a joint**?
   A. Dermatitis
   B. Arthritis
   C. Hepatitis
   D. Neuritis
5. The suffix **"-ectomy"** refers to:
   A. Cutting into
   B. Surgical repair
   C. Surgical removal
   D. Visual examination
6. A "gastroscopy" is best described as:
   A. Removal of the stomach
   B. Visual examination of the stomach
   C. Surgical repair of the stomach
   D. Inflammation of the stomach
7. The term **"tachycardia"** most closely means:
   A. Slow heart rate
   B. Fast heart rate
   C. Enlarged heart
   D. Heart pain
8. The term "dermatology" literally refers to:
   A. The study of bones
   B. The study of nerves
   C. The study of the skin
   D. The study of blood
9. In directional terms, **anterior** refers to:
   A. Back side
   B. Front side
   C. Above
   D. Below
10. The term **"lateral"** means:
    A. Toward the midline
    B. Away from the midline
    C. Above another structure
    D. On the surface
11. A patient with **myalgia** is experiencing:
    A. Muscle pain
    B. Bone fracture

C. Skin rash
D. Vision loss

12. The term "polyuria" most closely means:
A. Pain with urination
B. No urination
C. Excessive urination
D. Blood in urine
13. In the chart, "NPO after midnight" means the patient:
A. May only have clear liquids
B. May eat or drink freely
C. May have nothing by mouth after midnight
D. Should avoid medications after midnight
14. The abbreviation "PRN" in an order means:
A. At bedtime
B. As needed
C. Once a day
D. Before meals
15. "IM injection" refers to a medication given:
A. Into a vein
B. Under the skin
C. Into a muscle
D. By mouth
16. Which of the following abbreviations is considered **unsafe** or easily misread in many facilities?
A. PO
B. SubQ
C. U (for units)
D. IM
17. The safest way to write an order for 5 units of insulin is:
A. 5 U
B. 5 units
C. 5.0 U
D. 05 U
18. In documentation, "Pt c/o SOB x 2 days" most accurately means:
A. Patient complains of shortness of breath for two days
B. Patient has no shortness of breath
C. Patient sleeps well for two days
D. Patient has lower blood pressure for two days
19. The symbol "↑" next to BP in a note most likely means:
A. Blood pressure unchanged
B. Reduced blood pressure
C. Increased blood pressure
D. No blood pressure taken
20. Which documentation entry is the **most objective and professional**?
A. "The patient is annoying and noncompliant."

B. "The patient was lazy about taking meds."
C. "Patient states, 'I did not take my blood pressure medication today'; BP 168/96 mmHg."
D. "Patient doesn't care about health."

21. A patient asks what "hypertension" means. The CMA's **best** response is:
A. "It's just a big word; don't worry."
B. "It means your blood pressure is higher than normal."
C. "It means your heart is failing."
D. "It means you have heart cancer."
22. The term "leukocytosis" most likely refers to:
A. Low white blood cell count
B. High white blood cell count
C. Red blood cell disease
D. Blood clot in a vein
23. In the term "osteoporosis," the root "oste/o" means:
A. Joint
B. Muscle
C. Bone
D. Nerve
24. A provider writes an order using an abbreviation the CMA doesn't recognize. The CMA's **best** action is to:
A. Guess the meaning based on context
B. Look it up in a non-medical dictionary only
C. Clarify the abbreviation with the provider or approved reference before acting
D. Ignore it and skip the order
25. A patient is told they have "benign" test results. The most accurate plain-language explanation is:
A. "The results show cancer that will spread quickly."
B. "The results show a non-cancerous finding."
C. "The results are always fatal."
D. "The results mean we have no idea what's happening."

Answer Key – Chapter 11 (with Justifications)

1. **B** – "-megaly" means enlargement, so cardiomegaly is an enlarged heart.
2. **C** – "Hypo-" means below or low, as in low blood sugar (hypoglycemia).
3. **D** – "Hepat/o" refers to the liver, as in hepatitis (inflammation of the liver).
4. **B** – "Arthr/o" = joint and "-itis" = inflammation, so arthritis is joint inflammation.
5. **C** – "-ectomy" indicates surgical removal, such as appendectomy.
6. **B** – "-scopy" is visual examination; gastroscopy is visual examination of the stomach.
7. **B** – "Tachy-" = fast and "cardia" = heart; tachycardia is a fast heart rate.
8. **C** – "Dermat/o" = skin and "-logy" = study of; dermatology is the study of the skin.
9. **B** – Anterior means toward the front of the body.
10. **B** – Lateral means away from the midline, toward the side.
11. **A** – "My/o" = muscle and "-algia" = pain; myalgia is muscle pain.
12. **C** – "Poly-" = many/excessive and "-uria" relates to urine; polyuria is excessive urination.
13. **C** – NPO (nil per os) means nothing by mouth, so no food or drink after midnight.

14. **B** – PRN means “as needed,” often for symptom relief medications.
15. **C** – IM (intramuscular) injections go into a muscle.
16. **C** – “U” for units is easily misread and is on many “do-not-use” lists; safer to write “units.”
17. **B** – Writing “5 units” prevents confusion that “5 U” could be misread as “50” or similar.
18. **A** – “Pt c/o SOB x 2 days” translates to “patient complains of shortness of breath for two days.”
19. **C** – The up arrow (↑) indicates an increase; here, increased blood pressure.
20. **C** – This entry quotes the patient, provides specific BP data, and avoids judgmental language—making it objective and professional.
21. **B** – Hypertension means high blood pressure; this explanation is accurate and patient-friendly.
22. **B** – “Leuk/o” = white and “-cytosis” often indicates increased cells; leukocytosis is high white blood cell count.
23. **C** – “Oste/o” refers to bone, as in osteoporosis (porous bone).
24. **C** – Unfamiliar abbreviations must be clarified with the provider or approved resources; guessing is unsafe.
25. **B** – “Benign” means non-cancerous; it does not mean fatal or unknown.

Chapter 12

Medical Law, Ethics, and Professionalism

CMAs work at the intersection of clinical care, patient privacy, and professional behavior. Even when you're not the decision-maker, your actions must follow laws, ethical standards, and workplace policies. This chapter reviews the key legal and ethical concepts you're expected to know for the CMA exam and for safe, professional practice.

12.1 Legal Foundations: Scope of Practice and Delegation

YOUR **scope of practice** defines what you're legally allowed to do as a CMA in your state and under your credential. Providers and nurses may **delegate** certain tasks to you, but you must never step outside what the law and your training allow. The exam frequently checks whether you know when to act, when to assist, and when to say, "That's outside my scope."

- Scope of practice for the CMA
- Delegation and the CMA's responsibilities

Scope of practice describes the procedures, actions, and processes a CMA is permitted to perform under supervision, as determined by state law and facility policy. It typically includes tasks like taking vital signs, administering certain medications under orders, performing EKGs, collecting specimens, and patient education within guidelines. It does **not** include diagnosing, prescribing, independently changing treatment plans, or making high-level medical decisions. On the exam, if an option asks you to prescribe or alter doses on your own, that's a clear scope-of-practice violation.

Delegation occurs when a licensed provider or nurse assigns tasks to you that are within your capabilities and legal boundaries. Your responsibility is to accept only those tasks you're trained and competent to perform and to ask for clarification if an order is unclear. If you feel a task is unsafe or outside your scope, you must speak up respectfully. CMA exam questions often reward answers where you clarify, refuse unsafe delegation, or seek help rather than blindly doing something questionable.

12.2 Informed Consent and the Patient's Right to Refuse

PATIENTS HAVE THE RIGHT to understand what's being done to them and to agree—or refuse—before it happens. **Informed consent** is a legal and ethical requirement for many procedures and treatments. The CMA doesn't usually obtain consent but plays an important role in supporting the process.

- Elements of informed consent
- Patient's right to refuse treatment

Informed consent requires that the patient receive information about the nature of the procedure, its risks and benefits, alternatives, and likely outcomes of refusing. The provider typically explains this and answers questions, and the patient then agrees voluntarily—often in writing for more invasive procedures. As a CMA, you may witness signatures, verify that forms are complete, and ensure the correct patient is signing, but you do not alter or explain risks beyond your scope. On the exam, if a patient says they don't understand, the correct response is to inform the provider, not to "wing it" with your own medical explanation.

Patients also have the right to refuse treatments, procedures, or tests—even if their decision seems unwise. Your role is to respect that right, avoid pressuring or threatening them, and document the refusal according to policy. You should notify the provider whenever a patient refuses an important procedure or medication so it can be discussed further. CMA questions often test whether you honor a patient's refusal instead of forcing cooperation or falsifying records.

12.3 Confidentiality, HIPAA, and Protected Health Information (PHI)

PATIENT INFORMATION is private and must be protected. Laws like HIPAA (in the U.S.) set standards for how health information is used, disclosed, and stored. The CMA exam expects you to recognize what counts as PHI and how to keep it secure.

- Protected Health Information and confidentiality
- Appropriate vs. inappropriate sharing and access

Protected Health Information (PHI) includes any individually identifiable health information—names, addresses, birth dates, medical record numbers, diagnoses, or treatment details—whether in paper, electronic, or spoken form. Confidentiality means you only access or share PHI when it's necessary for patient care, payment, or operations and allowed by policy. This also applies to conversations; discussing patient details in public spaces like elevators or waiting rooms is not appropriate. On the exam, if you see a CMA chatting about patient diagnoses with friends, that's a clear HIPAA violation.

Appropriate sharing means giving information only to people who are authorized and have a legitimate need to know: the patient, involved healthcare providers, or others identified by the patient or law. Inappropriate sharing includes giving information to curious coworkers not involved in care, to family members without permission, or via unsecured channels like personal email or social media. You should also log out of EHRs when leaving a workstation and keep screens turned away from public view. CMA test questions almost always favor answers that protect privacy and seek clarification before releasing information.

12.4 Documentation, Medical Records, and Legal Protections

MEDICAL RECORDS SERVE as both a communication tool and a legal document. What you chart can be used to defend care—or to show that care was incomplete or negligent. The CMA must document carefully, honestly, and within policy.

- Principles of accurate, timely documentation
- Legal aspects of medical records and amendment rules

Accurate documentation includes recording facts, not opinions; using clear, specific language; and including date, time, and your credentials. Entries should be made as soon as possible after events occur, and late entries should be labeled as such per policy. You should never erase, obscure, or alter past entries in a way that hides errors. On exam questions, correct answers involve creating complete, factual notes rather than vague statements like "everything done."

Medical records are legal documents that may be requested in audits, lawsuits, or insurance reviews. If you make a mistake in documentation, you typically draw a single line through the error, label it as an error, add your initials and date, and then write the correct information—never white-out or delete. Patients have rights to access their records, but release is done through proper channels, not by casually printing and handing out information without authorization. The CMA exam favors options that treat documentation with seriousness and follow proper correction procedures.

12.5 Negligence, Malpractice, and Professional Liability

NEGLIGENCE AND MALPRACTICE involve failing to meet a standard of care, leading to patient harm. While CMAs aren't independently licensed like physicians, your actions can still contribute to legal liability. The exam tests basic understanding of these concepts and how to avoid risky behavior.

- Negligence and malpractice concepts
- Ways CMAs reduce legal risk

Negligence refers to failing to act with the care a reasonably prudent person would use in a similar situation, resulting in harm. Malpractice is a form of professional negligence by a healthcare provider that leads to patient injury. Examples include giving a medication ordered for a different patient, ignoring critical symptoms, or not following established procedures. On exam questions, unsafe shortcuts—like skipping identity checks or documentation—often signal negligent behavior.

CMAs reduce legal risk by following policies, staying within scope, asking for help when unsure, and documenting carefully. You should complete required training, keep skills up to date, and participate in safety programs such as incident reporting. If you see an error or near miss, reporting it according to policy helps prevent future harm and shows commitment to quality improvement. The CMA exam typically rewards answers that show proactive, safety-focused behavior rather than denial or cover-ups.

12.6 Ethics: Autonomy, Beneficence, Nonmaleficence, and Justice

ETHICS ARE MORAL PRINCIPLES that guide healthcare decisions, even beyond what the law strictly says. Four common principles are autonomy, beneficence, nonmaleficence, and justice. The CMA exam uses these ideas to frame questions about right vs. wrong choices in patient care.

- Respect for autonomy and beneficence
- Nonmaleficence ("do no harm") and justice

Autonomy means respecting a competent patient's right to make their own decisions, even when you disagree. Beneficence means acting in the patient's best interest—promoting their well-being and helping them. For example, educating a patient about their medications supports beneficence, while respecting their choice to decline a treatment supports autonomy. On the exam, answers that bully or trick patients into decisions generally violate autonomy and are wrong.

Nonmaleficence is the duty to avoid causing harm. This includes avoiding unnecessary procedures, double-checking medications, and reporting unsafe conditions. Justice involves fairness—treating patients equitably regardless of race, gender, income, or personal beliefs. The CMA must avoid discrimination and provide the same level of respect and effort for every patient. Exam questions often present subtle ethical conflicts where the best answer is the one that avoids harm and treats patients fairly while still respecting their choices.

12.7 Cultural Competence, Bias, and Professional Boundaries

HEALTHCARE HAPPENS in a culturally diverse setting, and your personal beliefs must not interfere with patient care. Cultural competence and bias awareness are essential for ethical, professional behavior. The CMA exam frequently tests whether you maintain boundaries and avoid discrimination.

- Cultural sensitivity and avoiding bias
- Professional boundaries with patients and coworkers

Cultural sensitivity involves recognizing that patients may have different beliefs about illness, treatments, family roles, and communication styles. You don't need to adopt their beliefs, but you must show respect, ask open questions, and avoid stereotyping. For example, instead of assuming a patient won't accept certain treatments, you ask what they prefer and share options. Exam scenarios often reward answers that seek understanding instead of judging or mocking cultural practices.

Professional boundaries mean keeping relationships with patients and coworkers appropriate and focused on care. You should not accept large personal gifts, date patients, or share overly personal details that blur roles. Social media adds complexity; posting about patients (even anonymously) or complaining about coworkers online can violate boundaries and confidentiality. On the CMA exam, answers that maintain respectful distance and protect privacy are correct, while those that cross into personal or romantic involvement are not.

12.8 Professional Behavior, Communication, and Teamwork

PROFESSIONALISM IS not just about knowledge; it's also about how you act, speak, and collaborate. The CMA often serves as a communication bridge between patients and the healthcare team. The exam includes many scenarios testing how you handle conflicts, feedback, and teamwork.

- Professional attitudes and behaviors in the workplace
- Effective communication and conflict resolution with the team

Professional behavior includes punctuality, appropriate attire, honesty, reliability, and a positive attitude toward learning and feedback. You should avoid gossip, rude comments, and disruptive behavior. When you make a mistake, acknowledging it and working to correct it is more professional than denying or blaming others. The exam tends to reward options that show humility, accountability, and respect.

Effective communication with coworkers involves active listening, clear and concise information sharing, and respect for others' roles. When conflicts arise, you should address them privately and calmly, focusing on patient care rather than personal grudges. If conflicts affect safety or cannot be resolved directly, involving a supervisor is appropriate. CMA exam questions generally favor answers where you address issues through proper channels instead of arguing in front of patients or spreading resentment.

12.9 Patient Rights, Advance Directives, and Special Situations

PATIENTS HAVE SPECIFIC rights, including privacy, informed consent, and participation in decisions. Some patients have advance directives that outline their wishes if they can't speak for themselves. The CMA must respect these documents and rights without making independent legal judgments.

- Basic patient rights and responsibilities
- Advance directives, DNR orders, and CMA's role

Patient rights include respectful treatment, privacy, access to information, participating in decisions, and the right to refuse care. Patients also have responsibilities, such as providing accurate information and following agreed treatment plans when possible. You may help by giving them written rights notices and answering basic questions within your scope. On the exam, choices that ignore expressed patient preferences usually conflict with these rights.

Advance directives (like living wills or durable powers of attorney for healthcare) express a patient's wishes about life-sustaining treatments if they become unable to decide. DNR (Do Not Resuscitate) orders or POLST forms may specify limits on resuscitation. The CMA does not create or override these documents but must be aware they exist and follow facility protocols when they apply. Exam questions often test whether you follow documented orders rather than ignoring them or acting based on personal beliefs.

12.10 Reporting Obligations, Incident Reports, and Whistleblowing

IN SOME SITUATIONS, CMAs are required to report concerns—for example, suspected abuse, certain diseases, or safety incidents. Reporting is not "snitching"; it's part of protecting patients and the public. The CMA exam checks whether you recognize these responsibilities and follow proper procedures.

- Incident reports and internal safety reporting
- Mandatory reporting (abuse, public health, and unsafe conditions)

Incident reports are internal documents used to record unusual events such as patient falls, medication errors, or near misses. They are factual, non-accusatory, and separate from the medical record. Completing an incident report helps the organization identify patterns and improve systems. On the exam, correct answers involve completing these forms honestly and promptly, not altering charts to hide what happened.

Mandatory reporting can include suspected child or elder abuse, certain communicable diseases, and unsafe or impaired coworkers, depending on laws and policies. As a CMA, you don't investigate or prove the problem; you document what you observed and notify the appropriate supervisor or authority. Failure to report can itself be a legal or ethical violation. Exam questions typically reward answers where you follow mandatory reporting laws and organizational policies to protect vulnerable people and public health.

Practice Questions – Chapter 12 (25 Questions)

THESE QUESTIONS FOCUS on scope of practice, informed consent and refusal, confidentiality/HIPAA, documentation, negligence, ethics, cultural competence, professionalism, patient rights, advance directives, and reporting.

1. A provider asks the CMA to "adjust the patient's insulin dose based on how they look today." The CMA's **best** response is to:
   A. Adjust the dose independently
   B. Refuse and tell the provider they are wrong
   C. State that changing doses is outside CMA scope and ask the provider to write a specific order
   D. Guess a dose that seems safe

2. Which situation best represents **informed consent**?
   A. The patient signs a form without any explanation
   B. The provider explains the procedure, risks, benefits, and alternatives, and the patient voluntarily agrees
   C. The CMA tells the patient they must sign or leave
   D. The caregiver signs without the patient knowing anything
3. A patient refuses a recommended injection after hearing the explanation. The CMA should:
   A. Force the injection because it's important
   B. Respect the refusal, document it, and notify the provider
   C. Give the injection secretly
   D. Argue loudly until the patient agrees
4. Which of the following is considered **Protected Health Information (PHI)**?
   A. Clinic's posted hours
   B. A patient's diagnosis and date of birth together
   C. Number of chairs in the waiting room
   D. The clinic's address
5. The CMA is discussing a patient's lab results with a friend at a restaurant. This is:
   A. Acceptable if no one is listening
   B. A breach of confidentiality/HIPAA
   C. Allowed if the friend is curious
   D. Required for learning
6. When accessing medical records, the CMA should:
   A. Access any chart out of curiosity
   B. Access only records needed to perform their job duties
   C. Look up charts for friends who ask
   D. Share login credentials with coworkers
7. The safest way to correct an error in a paper medical record is to:
   A. Erase it completely
   B. Use white-out so it isn't visible
   C. Draw a single line through the error, label it as an error, initial and date, and write the correct information
   D. Tear out the page and start over
8. Failing to identify a patient correctly and then giving them another patient's medication is an example of:
   A. Good teamwork
   B. Informed consent
   C. Negligence
   D. HIPAA compliance
9. Respecting a competent adult patient's decision to refuse a treatment, even when it might benefit them, reflects the ethical principle of:
   A. Justice
   B. Autonomy
   C. Beneficence
   D. Nonmaleficence
10. The ethical principle of **nonmaleficence** means:
   A. Doing good for others
   B. Treating everyone exactly the same

C. Avoiding harm to patients
D. Making decisions for patients

11. A CMA makes a medication error but notices it immediately and reports it according to policy. This action is:
A. Unprofessional and should be hidden
B. Professional and helps improve safety
C. Illegal in all cases
D. Only necessary if the patient is angry

12. A CMA says, "I don't like treating patients from that neighborhood; they never follow instructions." This comment shows:
A. Cultural competence
B. Appropriate humor
C. Bias and unprofessional attitude
D. Evidence-based practice

13. Which behavior best maintains **professional boundaries** with patients?
A. Accepting expensive personal gifts from a patient
B. Meeting a patient privately for dates
C. Being friendly and respectful while keeping the relationship focused on care
D. Sharing intimate personal problems with patients

14. A coworker repeatedly makes rude comments about a patient within earshot of others. The CMA's best response is to:
A. Join in the comments
B. Ignore it and laugh
C. Speak privately with the coworker or notify a supervisor if it continues, focusing on professionalism and respect
D. Post about it online

15. A patient asks to see their medical record. The CMA should:
A. Immediately hand over the chart without any process
B. Tell the patient they are never allowed to see it
C. Follow facility policy for record access and involve the appropriate department or provider
D. Read it aloud loudly in the waiting room

16. A DNR (Do Not Resuscitate) order is present in the patient's chart. In an arrest situation, the CMA should:
A. Ignore the DNR and start full CPR on their own
B. Follow facility policy regarding DNR orders and notify the provider/charge nurse immediately
C. Destroy the DNR form
D. Decide personally whether the order is right or wrong

17. Which scenario best demonstrates **objective documentation**?
A. "Patient is rude and difficult."
B. "The patient seems like a liar."
C. "Patient stated, 'I will not take that medication,' and refused after explanation; provider notified."
D. "A patient is a bad person."

18. A CMA witnesses what appears to be child abuse signs and suspects neglect. The most appropriate action is to:
A. Ignore it because it's private family business

B. Post anonymously on social media
C. Document observations objectively and follow mandatory reporting policy
D. Confront the suspected abuser in front of everyone

19. An incident report should be completed when:
A. A patient fall or medication error occurs, even if no one seems hurt
B. Everything goes perfectly
C. A staff member wants to complain about lunch options
D. A patient has a normal vital sign

20. A CMA posts on social media: "Crazy shift—our diabetic patient in Room 4 almost passed out again!" even without a name. This is:
A. Acceptable because no name is used
B. Unprofessional and potentially a confidentiality breach
C. Required for debriefing
D. Encouraged for learning

21. A patient is treated rudely by another staff member and complains to the CMA. The CMA should:
A. Say "That's just how they are, get used to it."
B. Ignore the complaint
C. Listen respectfully and follow facility process for reporting patient concerns, such as informing a supervisor
D. Tell the patient to file a lawsuit immediately

22. Justice in healthcare mainly refers to:
A. Giving more care to patients you like
B. Treating patients fairly and equitably
C. Always agreeing with the provider
D. Avoiding any documentation

23. During a heated disagreement with a nurse about responsibilities, the professional CMA response is to:
A. Argue loudly in front of patients
B. Gossip about the nurse to other staff
C. Discuss the issue privately, focusing on patient care, and involve a supervisor if needed
D. Refuse to speak to the nurse forever

24. A provider uses an unclear abbreviation in a medication order. For safety, the CMA should:
A. Guess its meaning and proceed
B. Clarify the order with the provider before the medication is given
C. Ask another patient
D. Ignore the order

25. A CMA notices the fire exit in a busy clinic is blocked by boxes. The most appropriate action is to:
A. Ignore it; it's not clinical
B. Move or arrange to move the boxes and report the safety hazard per policy
C. Wait until someone else notices
D. Stack more boxes to save space

Answer Key – Chapter 12 (with Justifications)

1. **C** – Adjusting insulin doses is outside CMA scope; the CMA should request a specific provider order rather

than changing doses independently.

2. **B** – Informed consent requires explanation of procedure, risks, benefits, and alternatives, followed by voluntary agreement.
3. **B** – Patients may refuse treatment; the CMA must respect the refusal, document it, and notify the provider.
4. **B** – A diagnosis plus date of birth clearly identifies a patient and is PHI.
5. **B** – Discussing patient information with a friend in public is a confidentiality/HIPAA breach.
6. **B** – CMAs should only access records necessary for their job tasks; curiosity access is prohibited.
7. **C** – Legal corrections are made by a single line, notation, initials, date, and correct information—never erasing or hiding.
8. **C** – Giving another patient's medication due to identification failure is negligent and can cause harm.
9. **B** – Autonomy is the ethical principle of respecting a patient's right to make their own decisions.
10. **C** – Nonmaleficence means "do no harm" and avoid causing injury or suffering.
11. **B** – Reporting errors promptly is professional and supports patient safety and quality improvement.
12. **C** – The statement shows bias and a negative attitude toward a group, which is unprofessional.
13. **C** – Maintaining a friendly but care-focused relationship respects professional boundaries.
14. **C** – Addressing rude comments privately or with a supervisor supports professionalism and respect.
15. **C** – Patients have rights to access records, but the process must follow facility policy and legal requirements.
16. **B** – DNR orders must be respected according to facility policy; CMAs should notify appropriate staff rather than ignore or destroy them.
17. **C** – This entry quotes the patient, describes specific behavior, and documents provider notification, making it objective and professional.
18. **C** – Suspected abuse requires objective documentation and mandatory reporting per law and policy.
19. **A** – Incident reports should be completed for falls, errors, or near misses, even without obvious injury.
20. **B** – Posting clinical situations on social media, even without names, is unprofessional and may violate confidentiality.
21. **C** – Listening respectfully and using formal complaint channels supports patient rights and professionalism.
22. **B** – Justice is about fair, equitable treatment of all patients, not favoritism.
23. **C** – Handling disagreements privately, focusing on patient care, and involving supervision as needed is professional.
24. **B** – Any unclear order must be clarified with the provider before medication is given to prevent errors.
25. **B** – Blocking fire exits is a hazard; removing/arranging removal and reporting supports safety and legal compliance.

Chapter 13

Integrated CMA Exam Review & Test-Taking Strategies

By this point in your prep, you've seen every major content area that appears on the CMA (AAMA) exam. Chapter 13 ties everything together so you can think like the exam: integrating clinical knowledge, administrative skills, communication, ethics, and professionalism into realistic scenarios. You'll also learn test-taking strategies to help you manage time, reduce anxiety, and avoid common traps on exam day.

13.1 Understanding the CMA Exam Structure and Expectations

KNOWING **how** the exam is built helps you understand what it's really asking from you. The CMA exam isn't just random trivia; it's designed to test safe, entry-level practice across domains. Understanding structure helps frame your study and reduce surprises on test day.

- Domains and the big-picture skill set being tested
- What "entry-level competent CMA" means in exam terms

The CMA exam is divided into major domains like Clinical, General, and Administrative, each covering multiple topics such as infection control, pharmacology, anatomy, communication, and office procedures. Questions often mix these areas—for example, a clinical scenario that also tests professionalism and documentation. The test is less about memorizing obscure facts and more about applying solid fundamentals across multiple situations. Thinking in terms of domains can help you identify your strong and weak areas during review.

"Entry-level competent CMA" means someone who can perform safely under supervision in a typical outpatient setting. The exam expects you to recognize dangerous situations, follow policies, stay within scope, and communicate effectively—not to act as a provider. When you're unsure, ask yourself: "What would a safe, newly certified CMA do here?" This mindset usually points you toward the best answer, especially in ethics, safety, and legal questions.

13.2 Building a Strategic Study Plan for Final Review

WITH THE EXAM APPROACHING, you need a realistic, focused plan rather than trying to cram everything at once. A strategic review targets your weaknesses while keeping strengths sharp. The goal is efficiency, not exhaustion.

- Identifying strengths and weaknesses by domain
- Structuring a weekly or final-countdown review schedule

Identifying strengths and weaknesses starts with honest reflection and, ideally, results from practice quizzes or chapter tests. If you're consistently missing questions on pharmacology or EKG basics, those domains deserve extra time. For strong areas, you still want light review, but you don't need to relearn everything from scratch. Making a simple checklist of domains with "Strong / Medium / Weak" labels can give you clarity on how to prioritize.

A good review schedule breaks your time into focused blocks—such as one day heavy on Clinical content, another on Administrative, and another on General. Within each block, you might spend part of the time re-reading key sections and part of the time doing practice questions. As you get closer to the exam, you can shift toward a more mixed, "randomized" review that simulates test conditions. Building in short breaks, sleep, and some flexibility helps you stay consistent without burning out.

13.3 Integrating Content: Thinking Across Systems and Topics

REAL EXAM SCENARIOS rarely live neatly in one chapter; they often blend infection control, anatomy, communication, and laws all at once. To succeed, you must practice connecting dots instead of treating topics as isolated. Integrated thinking is the bridge between studying and real-world clinical reasoning.

- Recognizing multi-domain questions and what they're really testing
- Using "anchor concepts" to navigate complex scenarios

Multi-domain questions might present a clinical vignette where a patient comes in with chest pain, and the question asks about vital signs interpretation, communication with the provider, or appropriate documentation. On the surface, it looks like a cardiovascular question, but it's also testing your understanding of scope, ethics, or procedure. Learning to ask yourself, "What is the *main* safety issue here?" helps you identify what the exam cares about most in the scenario.

Anchor concepts are big, reliable ideas that guide your decisions—such as patient safety first, scope of practice, infection control basics, and accurate documentation. When a question feels confusing, you can come back to these anchors: "What keeps the patient safest?" "What is within the CMA's role?" "How do I protect privacy and document correctly?" These anchors often eliminate obviously wrong answers and point you toward the one that best reflects safe, professional practice.

13.4 Clinical Reasoning in Scenarios: Safety, Scope, and Priorities

MANY CMA QUESTIONS are mini-stories where you decide what to do next. These aren't trick questions; they're asking whether you can recognize priorities, stay in your lane, and act logically. Developing a simple "mental checklist" helps you respond calmly and consistently.

- Identifying red flags and patient safety priorities
- Staying within scope while still taking meaningful action

Red flags include chest pain, shortness of breath, signs of stroke, anaphylaxis, severe bleeding, and sudden confusion or unresponsiveness. When a vignette includes these, your first thought should be: "This might be an emergency." From there, you prioritize calling for help, notifying the provider, activating emergency protocols, and monitoring the patient. Questions usually favor answers that respond immediately to danger, rather than doing routine tasks or paperwork first.

Staying within scope means you don't diagnose, prescribe, or alter treatment independently, even if you think you know what's wrong. Instead, you gather information, document accurately, initiate allowed first-aid or BLS steps if trained and appropriate, and communicate promptly with the provider. The exam wants to see you act as a strong, safe team member—not as a "mini-provider." When in doubt, pick the answer where you support care, communicate clearly, and do not overstep.

13.5 Medication and Math Awareness: Spotting Unsafe Orders

WHILE YOU MAY NOT BE doing heavy calculations on the exam, you still need basic dosing awareness and the ability to spot something that doesn't look right. Many medication questions combine pharmacology basics with safety and documentation. Your goal is to catch unsafe or unclear situations, not to act as a pharmacist.

- Recognizing red flags in medication orders and labels
- Using estimation and unit awareness to avoid calculation traps

Red flags include unclear abbreviations, missing routes or frequencies, doses that look unusually large or small for an age group, or medications that conflict with known allergies. If any order lacks critical details, the safe exam answer is to clarify with the provider before administering. Similarly, labels that don't match the order in name, strength, or form must not be used without double-checking. The CMA exam consistently rewards caution when it comes to medication safety.

Estimation and unit awareness help you catch "impossible" values, like doses that are 10 times larger due to misplaced decimals, or confusing mg vs. mcg. Even if you're not doing exact calculations, you should be able to tell when something feels grossly off for a typical adult or pediatric dose. If a question gives you choices that include obviously huge doses and one moderate, realistic choice, your estimating skills can point you toward the safer answer. Always choose the option that mentions double-checking and clarifying rather than guessing.

13.6 Interpreting Charts, EHR Entries, and Ordered Data

THE EXAM OFTEN PRESENTS information in tables, short chart notes, or EHR snippets. You might see vital sign trends, medication lists, or brief documentation and be asked what to do next. Learning to read these quickly and accurately is a key test-day skill.

- Reading trends in vitals, labs, and notes
- Identifying inconsistencies or missing information in documentation

Trends are more powerful than single values. For example, one mildly elevated blood pressure might be less concerning than a steady rise from normal to significantly high readings over several visits. If the chart shows repeated abnormal vital signs or new symptoms, your job is to notice the pattern and recognize that it needs provider attention. On the test, this often appears as "Which of the following findings should the CMA report immediately?"

Inconsistencies or gaps in documentation can be a clue that something is wrong—like a medication order in the chart with no corresponding administration record, or a lab result that doesn't match the documented diagnosis. The exam expects you to notice when information is incomplete or contradictory and to respond by clarifying, not by guessing. You should also recognize when chart entries are too vague ("patient fine") and mentally replace them with more specific, objective phrasing.

13.7 Ethics, Communication, and "Most Appropriate Response" Questions

SOME OF THE TRICKIEST questions don't ask for facts, but for the **best** or **most appropriate** response to a situation. These often involve communication with patients or coworkers, ethical dilemmas, or professional behavior. Practice spotting the difference between technically possible and professionally best.

- Choosing responses that reflect empathy, respect, and clarity
- Balancing honesty, scope, and patient autonomy in communication

Empathic responses acknowledge feelings, show respect, and offer clear next steps. For example, when a patient is scared or upset, the best answer usually starts with "I understand this is difficult" or "It's normal to feel that way," followed by concrete support like offering to explain more or informing the provider. Answers that minimize ("You're overreacting"), joke inappropriately, or blame the patient are almost never correct on the exam.

Balancing honesty and scope means giving truthful, plain-language explanations without stepping into provider territory. If a patient asks, "Do I have cancer?" The CMA answer should direct them to the provider for interpretation, while still being kind and supportive. Likewise, respecting autonomy means accepting refusal of tests or treatment, documenting it, and notifying the provider—not tricking or pressuring the patient. The exam will almost always favor the response that is honest, respectful, and within your role.

13.8 Time Management and Pacing During the Exam

EVEN IF YOU KNOW THE content, poor time management can hurt your score. The CMA exam includes many questions, and spending too long on a few can leave others unanswered. Developing a simple pacing strategy can help you stay calm and efficient.

- Using a "first pass / second pass" approach
- Preventing perfectionism from slowing you down

A "first pass" approach means answering all the questions you feel reasonably confident about and marking the more difficult or time-consuming ones to revisit later. This ensures you collect as many points as possible from the questions you do know before spending extra time elsewhere. On your "second pass," you return to the marked items and think more deeply or perform any necessary calculations. This strategy can dramatically reduce the pressure of getting stuck early.

Perfectionism and overthinking can tempt you to reread the same question ten times. Remind yourself that standardized exams are not looking for the *perfect* answer, just the best choice among four. If you can eliminate one or two options quickly, you've already improved your odds. Setting informal time checkpoints—such as roughly where you should be halfway through—helps you notice if you're falling behind and need to move a little faster.

13.9 Multiple-Choice Strategy: Eliminating Distractors and Avoiding Traps

MULTIPLE-CHOICE EXAMS use distractor options to test whether you truly understand the material. You can often improve your score simply by becoming better at eliminating wrong answers. Knowing common trap patterns helps you avoid them on test day.

- Systematically ruling out clearly incorrect options
- Recognizing common trap patterns and extreme or unsafe answers

Ruling out wrong answers starts with identifying anything that violates basic safety, scope of practice, or clear facts. If an option involves ignoring chest pain, sharing PHI casually, or adjusting medications on your own, it's almost certainly wrong. Among the remaining options, compare each to your anchor concepts: which one best protects safety, respects rights, and follows policy? Even if you're unsure, eliminating obvious mistakes improves your chances.

Trap answers often look appealing because they mention something you studied—but they don't address the actual question or they add an unsafe twist. Be careful with options that use absolute words like "always" and "never," especially when they conflict with patient autonomy or clinical judgment. Some distractors sound dramatic but ignore the simpler, safer step (like notifying the provider). When in doubt, reread the question stem and ask, "What is this **really** asking me to decide?"

13.10 Exam Day Preparation, Anxiety Management, and Mindset

CONTENT AND STRATEGY matter, but so does your mental and physical state on exam day. Anxiety is normal, but you can keep it at manageable levels with basic preparation and self-care. Your mindset can turn the exam from a threat into a challenge you're ready to meet.

- Practical exam-day preparation and routines
- Managing anxiety and maintaining a confident, realistic mindset

Practical preparation includes knowing your test location and time, bringing required IDs, and arriving early to avoid last-minute stress. The night before, light review of key formulas or concepts is fine, but heavy cramming often backfires; prioritize sleep, hydration, and a reasonable meal. On the morning of the exam, give yourself enough time to settle in, breathe, and mentally review your anchor concepts: safety, scope, documentation, and professionalism.

To manage anxiety, use simple techniques like slow, deep breathing and anchoring thoughts: "I've prepared; I just need to do one question at a time." When you hit a difficult problem, mark it, move on, and remind yourself that no single question determines your outcome. A realistic mindset acknowledges that you won't feel 100% certain on every item—and that's okay. The CMA exam is about overall competence; by combining solid knowledge, smart strategies, and calm persistence, you maximize your chances of success.

CMA (AAMA) Mock Exam – 200 Questions

Instructions:

Choose the **one best answer** for each question.

1.

A PATIENT ARRIVES FOR a fasting blood draw and says, "I had coffee with cream 2 hours ago." The CMA's **best** action is to:

A. Proceed and ignore it
B. Proceed but say nothing
C. Inform the provider or lab and ask if the test should be rescheduled or noted as non-fasting
D. Cancel all future labs

2.

WHICH OF THE FOLLOWING tasks is **within** the CMA scope in most outpatient settings?

A. Prescribing antibiotics
B. Changing insulin doses based on judgment
C. Administering a provider-ordered IM injection per policy
D. Diagnosing hypertension

3.

THE PATIENT'S CHART lists a **severe penicillin allergy**. The provider orders amoxicillin. The CMA should:

A. Give it as ordered
B. Clarify the order with the provider before dispensing or administering
C. Delete the allergy from the chart
D. Substitute a different antibiotic

4.

WHICH OF THE FOLLOWING represents **subjective** data?

A. Temperature 101.2°F
B. "I feel dizzy when I stand up."
C. Pulse 88 bpm
D. O_2 saturation 95%

5.

THE **most appropriate** way to verify patient identity before venipuncture is:

A. Ask, "Are you Mr. Smith?"
B. Ask the patient to state full name and date of birth and compare to the order
C. Identify the patient by appearance only
D. Check with the person in the waiting room

6.

TO PREVENT SPECIMEN mislabeling, the CMA should:

A. Pre-label tubes before seeing the patient
B. Label tubes immediately after collection in the patient's presence
C. Label all specimens at the end of the shift
D. Have patients label their own tubes

7.

CLEAR TAPPING SOUNDS are first heard at 138 mmHg and disappear at 82 mmHg. The correct blood pressure to document is:

A. 138/82 mmHg
B. 82/138 mmHg
C. 138/80 mmHg
D. 120/80 mmHg

8.

WHICH ACTION **breaks sterile technique** during a minor procedure?

A. Keeping sterile items above waist level
B. Turning your back on the sterile field
C. Discarding items that fall below the waist
D. Opening sterile packs so contents drop onto the field

9.

DURING VENIPUNCTURE, the patient becomes pale and says, "I feel like I'm going to faint." The CMA should first:

A. Continue drawing to finish quickly
B. Stop the draw, release tourniquet, remove needle, assist to a safe position
C. Ignore the complaint
D. Ask the patient to stand

10.

AN UNLABELED URINE specimen is found on the counter. The correct action is to:

A. Guess which patient it belongs to
B. Label it with the only name you recall
C. Discard per policy and have a new specimen collected
D. Send it to the lab unlabeled

11.

WHICH FINDING IS **most urgent** to report to the provider?

A. BP 134/82 in adult
B. Temp 99.4°F (37.4°C)
C. New chest pain with shortness of breath

D. Mild ankle swelling after working all day

12.

PROPER INSTRUCTIONS for a clean-catch midstream urine sample include:

A. "No cleaning is needed."
B. "Collect only the very first drops."
C. "Start urinating into the toilet, then move the cup into the stream without touching inside."
D. "Fill the cup to the very top."

13.

A PATIENT CALLS ASKING for lab results. The CMA should:

A. Read all results with no verification
B. Confirm identity and follow office policy, involving the provider as required
C. Refuse to talk to them
D. Post results online

14.

WHICH BEST DESCRIBES **Protected Health Information (PHI)**?

A. Only written charts
B. Any individually identifiable health information in any form
C. Only billing information
D. Only lab results

15.

INFORMED CONSENT MEANS:

A. Patient signs a form without explanation
B. Provider explains procedure, risks, benefits, alternatives, and patient voluntarily agrees
C. CMA demands the patient sign
D. Family signs without the patient knowing

16.

A PROVIDER ORDER READS "10 U insulin SC now." The CMA recognizes "U" is unsafe and should:

A. Change it to "10 units" without asking
B. Clarify and have provider rewrite as "10 units" before giving
C. Assume it means 100 units
D. Ignore and proceed

17.

THE CMA ASKS ABOUT medications. The patient lists prescriptions, OTCs, and herbal supplements. The CMA should:

A. Record prescriptions only
B. Record all substances and alert the provider to review for interactions

C. Tell the patient supplements don't matter
D. Tell the patient to stop everything

18.

WHEEZING AND DIFFICULTY exhaling primarily involve which system?
A. Digestive
B. Respiratory
C. Musculoskeletal
D. Integumentary

19.

"POLYURIA" MEANS:
A. No urine
B. Painful urination
C. Excessive urination
D. Blood in urine

20.

A TODDLER HAS A RECTAL temp of 104.2°F (40.1°C), is lethargic, and not drinking. The CMA should:
A. Consider this mild and give routine advice
B. Notify the provider immediately
C. Send home with no follow-up
D. Record as normal

21.

AN EKG TRACING SHOWS wandering baseline due to loose electrodes. The CMA should:
A. Ignore it and file as normal
B. Reposition/secure electrodes and repeat
C. Diagnose myocardial infarction
D. Throw it away and do nothing

22.

WHICH BMI-RELATED TASK is appropriate for the CMA?
A. Diagnosing obesity
B. Using height/weight to calculate BMI and entering it for provider review
C. Prescribing diet medications
D. Changing insulin dosing

23.

THE ROUTE ABBREVIATION **PO** means:
A. Intramuscular
B. Intravenous

C. By mouth
D. Rectal

24.

AN OLDER ADULT WHO was previously alert now appears confused. The CMA should:
A. Assume it's normal aging
B. Document and notify the provider
C. Tell the patient to focus
D. Refuse to proceed

25.

WHICH DOCUMENTATION is most **objective**?
A. "The patient is lazy."
B. "The patient is rude."
C. "Patient stated, 'I won't take that pill,' and refused medication after explanation; provider notified."
D. "The patient doesn't care about health."

26.

A PATIENT WITH DIABETES is pale, shaky, sweaty, and says they feel weak. This most likely suggests:
A. Hyperglycemia
B. Hypoglycemia
C. Normal status
D. Ear infection

27.

AN APPROPRIATE SUBCUTANEOUS injection site for an adult is:
A. Over the patella
B. Abdomen at least 2 inches from the umbilicus
C. Directly over the spine
D. Tip of the finger

28.

FOR VENIPUNCTURE WITH expected blood exposure, which PPE is typically required?
A. Gloves
B. N95 respirator only
C. Gown only
D. None

29.

A PATIENT SAYS, "I don't want my spouse to know my test results." The CMA should:
A. Promise to tell the spouse anyway
B. Explain that information is confidential and won't be shared without permission, consistent with law/policy

C. Call the spouse immediately
D. Refuse to care for the patient

30.

WHICH SCENARIO IS AN example of **negligence**?
A. Double-checking patient ID and meds
B. Failing to raise side rails for a toddler, who falls from the exam table
C. Washing hands before and after patient contact
D. Documenting care promptly

31.

A PARENT REPORTS THEIR 2-year-old is not using any words yet. The CMA should:
A. Ignore it; all children are different
B. Document as possible developmental delay and notify provider
C. Tell the parent they're overreacting
D. Diagnose autism

32.

A PATIENT SCHEDULED for a pelvic exam is tearful and anxious. The CMA's best response is:
A. "There's nothing to be scared of; relax."
B. "It's understandable to feel nervous. I'll explain each step and protect your privacy."
C. "If you're scared, we should cancel."
D. "You shouldn't feel that way."

33.

THE CMA IS ASKED TO perform a procedure they were never trained to do. The **best** action is:
A. Attempt it anyway
B. Politely explain they are untrained and request guidance or training
C. Lie and say they know how
D. Have the patient do it

34.

"QID" IN A MEDICATION order means:
A. Once daily
B. Twice daily
C. Three times daily
D. Four times daily

35.

A PREGNANT PATIENT reports severe headache, hand/face swelling, and visual changes. The CMA should:
A. Treat as normal pregnancy symptoms
B. Document and notify provider immediately

C. Tell patient to rest and ignore it
D. Delay report until next visit

36.

WHEN A PROVIDER USES an unclear abbreviation in an order, the CMA should:
A. Guess the meaning
B. Ask another patient
C. Clarify with the provider before acting
D. Ignore the order

37.

A PATIENT ASKS, "DO I have cancer from these lab results?" The CMA's best reply is:
A. "Yes, definitely."
B. "No, you're fine."
C. "The provider will review these results with you; I'll let them know you have questions."
D. "Expect the worst."

38.

THE CMA SUSTAINS A needle with a used needle. The **first** step is to:
A. Ignore it
B. Wash the area with soap and water and follow exposure protocol
C. Hide the incident
D. Wait for symptoms

39.

STANDARD (UNIVERSAL) precautions mean:
A. Using PPE only with known infections
B. Applying appropriate PPE with all patients based on anticipated exposure
C. Using gloves only if blood is visible
D. Reusing gloves between patients

40.

A PATIENT COLLAPSES in the waiting room, unresponsive with abnormal breathing. The CMA should first:
A. Check responsiveness and breathing, call for help, activate emergency response
B. Search for insurance card
C. Wait to see if they wake up
D. Finish paperwork

41.

AN OLDER ADULT WALKS unsteadily and holds onto furniture. The CMA should:
A. Laugh about it
B. Document and notify provider of possible fall risk

C. Ignore it
D. Refuse to assist

42.

WHICH TERM MEANS **inflammation of the liver**?
A. Nephritis
B. Hepatitis
C. Gastritis
D. Dermatitis

43.

"BRADYCARDIA" REFERS to:
A. Fast heart rate
B. Slow heart rate
C. Irregular blood pressure
D. No pulse

44.

WHICH DOCUMENTATION is best for a dressing change?
A. "Changed dressing."
B. "Everything looks okay."
C. "Dressing changed to left forearm laceration at 0930; wound cleansed with NS; sterile gauze applied; patient tolerated well."
D. "Arm looked gross."

45.

A PATIENT PRESENTS with facial droop, slurred speech, and arm weakness. The CMA should:
A. Give water and watch them
B. Have them wait for a routine appointment
C. Recognize possible stroke and notify provider/activate emergency response per protocol
D. Send them home

46.

A PATIENT'S BP HAS increased from 126/78 to 168/102 today. The CMA should:
A. Change the value to match previous readings
B. Document and promptly notify the provider
C. Ignore it
D. Tell the patient not to worry

47.

THE CMA DISCOVERED that epinephrine in the emergency kit expired last month. The appropriate action is:
A. Ignore it

B. Replace according to policy and report the issue
C. Use it first to avoid waste
D. Scratch out the expiration date

48.

"CHOLECYSTECTOMY" MEANS:
A. Inflammation of gallbladder
B. Surgical removal of gallbladder
C. Incision into gallbladder
D. Endoscopic view of gallbladder

49.

A PATIENT IS ANGRY about wait time and is speaking loudly. The CMA should:
A. Yell back
B. Remain calm, acknowledge frustration, and explain what can be done
C. Ignore them
D. Tell them to leave

50.

A CHILD HAS BRUISES in different stages of healing and vague caregiver explanations. The CMA should:
A. Ignore it
B. Document objectively and follow mandatory reporting policies
C. Post anonymously online
D. Confront caregiver loudly

51.

A PATIENT IS ABOUT to sign a surgical consent and says, "I don't really understand what they're going to do." The CMA should:
A. Tell them to sign anyway
B. Provide detailed risk counseling beyond scope
C. Notify the provider so they can re-explain before signing
D. Sign for the patient

52.

THE SAFEST WAY TO INDICATE "once a day" in an order is:
A. QD
B. OD
C. Daily
D. QOD

53.

THE LAB CALLS WITH a **critical potassium** value. The CMA should:

A. Say “okay” and hang up
B. Document, read back the result, and immediately notify provider
C. Wait until the end of the day
D. Tell other patients about it

54.

A PATIENT ASKS, “WHY do I need vaccines if I’m healthy?” The best response is:
A. “You don’t if you’re healthy.”
B. “Vaccines help your immune system prevent serious diseases and protect others around you.”
C. “We only give them money to make money.”
D. “They’re just for very sick people.”

55.

WHICH INSTRUCTION BEST supports medication adherence?
A. “Take it whenever you remember.”
B. “Follow the schedule on the label; if you miss a dose, call us or the pharmacist rather than doubling up.”
C. “Stop as soon as you feel better, even if not told to.”
D. “Change the dose if you feel like it’s too strong.”

56.

A CMA BECOMES AWARE a coworker is working while impaired by substances. The most appropriate action is to:
A. Ignore it
B. Joke about it
C. Report concerns through proper chain of command per policy
D. Post online

57.

THE “FIGHT OR FLIGHT” response is controlled mainly by the:
A. Parasympathetic nervous system
B. Sympathetic nervous system
C. Digestive system
D. Integumentary system

58.

WHICH ACTION SHOWS **cultural sensitivity**?
A. Assuming all patients from a culture share the same beliefs
B. Asking how the patient prefers information shared and who should be included in decisions
C. Refusing care to certain cultural groups
D. Making jokes about cultural practices

59.

TEACHING METERED-DOSE inhaler use for COPD, the CMA should:

A. Tell the patient to use it however they want
B. Demonstrate technique as instructed, then have patient return-demonstrate
C. Change the medication if they cough
D. Prescribe a different inhaler

60.

AT THE END OF A VISIT, a patient says, "I'm overwhelmed by everything I heard." The CMA should respond:
A. "You're overreacting."
B. "I understand this is a lot. Let's review the key points and I'll show you how to reach us with questions."
C. "That's your problem."
D. "You should have listened better."

61.

STANDARD PRECAUTIONS are used:
A. Only for patients with known infections
B. For all patients, based on anticipated exposure
C. Only in the hospital
D. Only if PPE is available

62.

WHICH IS AN EXAMPLE of **droplet precautions**?
A. Gloves only
B. Surgical mask when within 3–6 feet of a coughing patient
C. N95 for all patients
D. No precautions

63.

THE MAIN PURPOSE OF **hand hygiene** is to:
A. Protect the floor
B. Reduce transmission of microorganisms
C. Keep hands moisturized
D. Avoid glove use

64.

WHICH OF THE FOLLOWING is a **vector** in infection transmission?
A. Contaminated water
B. Coughing
C. Mosquito
D. Air current

65.

WHICH IS THE **minimum** time recommended for alcohol-based hand rub friction (per common guidelines)?

A. 2 seconds
B. 5 seconds
C. 15–20 seconds
D. 1 minute

66.

A CONTAMINATED NEEDLE should be disposed of in:

A. Regular trash
B. Biohazard bag
C. Sharps container
D. Recycling bin

67.

THE **primary** reason to perform quality control (QC) on POCT devices is to:

A. Save test strips
B. Ensure accuracy and reliability of patient results
C. Make the machine look busy
D. Avoid using labs

68.

A RAPID STREP TEST should be read at 5 minutes. Reading it at 20 minutes can:

A. Improve accuracy
B. Cause false results
C. Have no effect
D. Cancel the test automatically

69.

THE **first** step in the chain of infection is:

A. Susceptible host
B. Reservoir
C. Infectious agent
D. Mode of transmission

70.

WHICH VITAL SIGN CHANGE is most concerning?

A. BP from 118/72 to 120/74
B. Pulse from 76 to 80
C. Respirations from 18 to 28 with dyspnea
D. Temp from 98.6°F to 99.0°F

71.

FOR AN ADULT, THE **normal** resting respiratory rate is approximately:

A. 6–8 breaths per minute
B. 12–20 breaths per minute
C. 20–30 breaths per minute
D. 30–40 breaths per minute

72.

WHICH PULSE SITE IS commonly used for routine adult pulse checks?
A. Carotid
B. Radial
C. Popliteal
D. Dorsalis pedis

73.

BMI IS CALCULATED USING:
A. Weight only
B. Height only
C. Height and weight
D. Waist circumference only

74.

A PATIENT WITH ASTHMA is short of breath, using accessory muscles, and can only speak one–two words at a time. The CMA should:
A. Document and continue routine care
B. Recognize severe distress and notify provider/activate emergency protocols
C. Offer water only
D. Tell patient to walk more

75.

THE CENTRAL NERVOUS system consists of:
A. Brain and spinal cord
B. Brain and peripheral nerves
C. Spinal cord and autonomic nerves
D. Heart and lungs

76.

THE THYROID GLAND PRIMARILY regulates:
A. Blood clotting
B. Metabolism
C. Urinary output
D. Skin temperature only

77.

MOST NUTRIENT ABSORPTION occurs in the:

A. Stomach
B. Small intestine
C. Large intestine
D. Esophagus

78.

THE KIDNEYS' MAIN FUNCTIONS include:

A. Pumping blood
B. Filtering blood and forming urine
C. Producing bile
D. Storing feces

79.

"ERYTHEMA" MEANS:

A. Blue discoloration
B. Redness
C. Yellow discoloration
D. Blackening

80.

LIGAMENTS CONNECT:

A. Bone to bone
B. Muscle to bone
C. Muscle to muscle
D. Skin to bone

81.

WHICH OF THESE IS **most** likely to indicate infection at a wound?

A. Pale, cool skin
B. Redness, warmth, swelling, and purulent drainage
C. Slight bruising only
D. Dry, intact skin

82.

WHICH POSITION IS COMMONLY used for a rectal temperature in a small child?

A. Supine
B. Sims' or side-lying
C. Trendelenburg
D. Prone on stomach only

83.

FOR AN ADULT IM INJECTION in the deltoid, the needle length is typically:

A. 1–1.5 inches (depending on size)
B. 3 inches
C. ¼ inch
D. 5 inches

84.

A VACCINE DOSE HAS been left out of the fridge overnight. The CMA should:

A. Return it to fridge and use later
B. Freeze it to "reset"
C. Follow policy—do not use; consider it compromised
D. Use quickly before it warms more

85.

AFTER A VACCINE, EXPECTED **mild** reactions may include:

A. Anaphylaxis
B. Soreness at injection site and low-grade fever
C. Severe facial swelling
D. Inability to breathe

86.

WHICH INFORMATION MUST be documented after administering a vaccine?

A. Patient's favorite color
B. Vaccine name, lot number, manufacturer, dose, route, site, date
C. Weather conditions
D. Staff lunch plan

87.

INFORMED REFUSAL (PATIENT declines care) should be:

A. Ignored
B. Documented clearly and communicated to the provider
C. Met with threats
D. Overridden

88.

AN ADVANCE DIRECTIVE generally:

A. Gives instructions about care if the patient cannot decide
B. Is a type of infection record
C. Replaces all consent forms
D. Must be ignored by staff

89.

A DNR ORDER MEANS:

A. Do Not Reschedule
B. Do Not Resuscitate
C. Do Not Refer
D. Do Not Record

90.

WHICH IS THE **best** way to handle a conflict with a coworker?

A. Yell in front of patients
B. Gossip with other staff
C. Discuss privately, focusing on patient care, and involve supervisor if needed
D. Refuse to speak to them

91.

WHICH BEHAVIOR BEST supports professional boundaries?

A. Dating a current patient
B. Accepting expensive gifts from a patient
C. Being friendly but keeping the relationship focused on care
D. Sharing intimate personal problems with patients

92.

AN INCIDENT REPORT is completed to:

A. Punish staff
B. Document unusual events/falls/errors to improve safety
C. Replace the medical record
D. Blame patients

93.

"C/O" IN DOCUMENTATION means:

A. Can offer
B. Complains of
C. Care of
D. Check off

94.

"SOB" IN CLINICAL NOTES stands for:

A. Short of breath
B. Statement of benefits
C. Son of brother
D. Sign of bacteria

95.

“HYPERGLYCEMIA” REFERS to:

A. Low blood sugar
B. High blood sugar
C. High blood pressure
D. Low heart rate

96.

“GASTRITIS” MEANS:

A. Stomach inflammation
B. Joint inflammation
C. Brain tumor
D. Liver failure

97.

“NEPHRECTOMY” IS:

A. Kidney inflammation
B. Kidney removal
C. Kidney biopsy
D. Kidney x-ray

98.

A PATIENT ASKS WHAT “benign tumor” means. The CMA’s best plain-language explanation is:

A. “A non-cancerous growth.”
B. “An aggressive cancer.”
C. “Always fatal.”
D. “No idea what it is.”

99.

WHICH ABBREVIATION is on many “do not use” lists?

A. PO
B. IM
C. U (for units)
D. PRN

100.

WHEN DOCUMENTING, IF an error is made in a paper chart, the CMA should:

A. Erase it
B. Use white-out
C. Draw a single line through, mark as error, initial/date, and correct
D. Tear out the page

101.

A PATIENT DEMANDS TO know the exact cost of every test you're scheduling. The CMA's best response is to:

A. Guess an amount
B. Refuse to address costs
C. Provide available cost information or direct them to billing/insurance resources per policy
D. Tell them cost doesn't matter

102.

THE MAIN PURPOSE OF **triage** in an office setting is to:

A. Give diagnoses over the phone
B. Prioritize patients based on urgency of symptoms
C. Schedule based on who pays the most
D. Choose favorite patients

103.

WHICH TELEPHONE BEHAVIOR is most professional?

A. Speaking loudly and quickly
B. Answering with clinic name and your name, then asking how you can help
C. Saying "Yeah?"
D. Ignoring calls

104.

A PATIENT WANTS TO update their address and phone number. The CMA should:

A. Refuse to change it
B. Update demographic information in the EHR accurately
C. Change their diagnosis
D. Ignore the request

105.

WHICH SCHEDULING METHOD keeps patients booked at the same time, then seen in order of arrival?

A. Wave scheduling
B. Double booking
C. Open hours
D. Stream scheduling

106.

"STREAM SCHEDULING" generally means:

A. No appointments, walk-ins only
B. Patients scheduled at specific, evenly spaced times
C. All patients at the same time
D. Only emergency visits

107.

THE PRIMARY PURPOSE of a **tickler file/reminder system** is to:

A. Track staff birthdays
B. Provide reminders of future tasks, follow-ups, or due services
C. Store emergency supplies
D. Replace medical records

108.

WHICH COLLECTION STEP is appropriate when a patient can't pay a copay today?

A. Yell at them
B. Provide information on payment options according to policy and document discussion
C. Tear up their chart
D. Refuse to schedule future visits automatically

109.

A CLAIM IS **rejected** due to missing information. The CMA's role is to:

A. Ignore it
B. Correct or supply missing data and resubmit according to policy
C. Close the patient's account
D. Bill the provider personally

110.

PHI CAN BE FAXED WHEN:

A. The patient insists, with no other planning
B. It is sent to a correct, verified number using a cover sheet and policy is followed
C. The CMA is curious
D. It's convenient, regardless of destination

111.

WHICH IS APPROPRIATE for a patient sign-in sheet under privacy rules?

A. Full reason for visit listed publicly
B. Only name and appointment time per policy
C. Full SSN displayed
D. Diagnosis listed

112.

A CMA RECEIVES A SUBPOENA for medical records. The correct action is to:

A. Throw it away
B. Immediately hand over original chart without review
C. Notify the provider/office manager and follow legal/records policy
D. Call the news

113.

A PATIENT BECOMES VERBALLY abusive and threatens staff. The CMA should:

A. Respond with equal aggression
B. Leave them alone in a room
C. Follow clinic policy for disruptive patients, ensure safety, and notify supervisor/provider/security as required
D. Ignore the behavior

114.

WHICH IS THE **best** way to ask for a co-pay?

A. "You better pay or else."
B. "Your copay today is $20. How would you like to take care of that?"
C. "Pay if you feel like it."
D. "We don't really need it."

115.

A PATIENT WANTS A COPY of their medical record. The CMA should:

A. Refuse
B. Give the chart with no process
C. Follow policy for record release, including written request and any fees, and route to records staff
D. Tell them to pay cash under the table

116.

AN ELDERLY PATIENT doesn't understand a complex form. The CMA should:

A. Read it verbatim very quickly
B. Explain sections in plain language and offer to get the provider for clinical questions, without giving legal advice
C. Tell them to sign without reading
D. Refuse to help

117.

AN ERROR IS MADE IN a financial ledger. Proper correction should:

A. Be erased completely
B. Have a single line through the error with correction and initials/date
C. Be hidden
D. Not be corrected at all

118.

A PATIENT ARRIVES 30 minutes late for their appointment. The CMA should:

A. Automatically refuse to see them
B. Yell at them
C. Follow office policy, which may include asking the provider if they can still be seen or rescheduled
D. Close their chart forever

119.

THE MAIN PURPOSE OF a **reference (diagnostic) code** like ICD is to:

A. Track staff performance
B. Classify diagnoses for billing and statistics
C. Replace medications
D. Record vital signs

120.

CPT CODES ARE PRIMARILY used to:

A. Code diagnoses
B. Code procedures and services
C. Record vital signs
D. Track staff attendance

121.

WHICH IS AN EXAMPLE of a **modifier** in coding?

A. Adding one digit to change a diagnosis
B. A two-digit code that provides extra detail, such as bilateral procedure
C. Writing notes in the margin
D. Changing provider name

122.

WHICH COUGH SYMPTOM is more urgent to report in a patient with recent surgery?

A. Mild, dry cough
B. Cough with bright red blood
C. Occasional throat clearing
D. Morning cough only

123.

A PATIENT WITH DIABETES states they sometimes skip insulin doses to avoid weight gain. The CMA should:

A. Agree with skipping doses
B. Explain that insulin should not be changed without provider input and notify the provider of the concern
C. Ignore it
D. Tell them to stop insulin completely

124.

A PATIENT DOES NOT speak English well. The **best** strategy is:

A. Rely on children to interpret complex information
B. Use a qualified medical interpreter or language service per policy
C. Speak louder
D. Avoid giving information

125.

WHICH IS AN APPROPRIATE use of teach-back?

A. Asking, "Do you understand?"
B. Having the patient repeat instructions in their own words to confirm understanding
C. Giving written materials only
D. Quizzing the patient aggressively

126.

A PATIENT REFUSES TO sign an ABN (Advance Beneficiary Notice) for a service that may not be covered. The CMA should:

A. Force them to sign
B. Document refusal and follow office/insurer policy on whether service can proceed
C. Forge signature
D. Ignore the form

127.

THE **primary** purpose of OSHA regulations in healthcare is to:

A. Protect patients financially
B. Protect workers from workplace hazards and exposure
C. Regulate billing
D. Set malpractice premiums

128.

WHICH IS AN EXAMPLE of an engineering control for bloodborne pathogens?

A. Handwashing
B. Safety-engineered needles
C. Staff training
D. PPE use

129.

THE EXPOSURE CONTROL plan must be:

A. Secret
B. Written and accessible to employees
C. Optional
D. Verbal only

130.

"AUTONOMY" IN ETHICS refers to:

A. Doing good
B. Doing no harm
C. Fairness
D. Respecting patients' right to make their own decisions

131.

"BENEFICENCE" MEANS:

A. Doing good and promoting patient welfare
B. Doing nothing
C. Always doing what's cheapest
D. Keeping secrets only

132.

"JUSTICE" IN HEALTHCARE primarily means:

A. Always siding with the provider
B. Treating patients fairly and equitably
C. Avoiding documentation
D. Sharing information online

133.

WHICH IS AN EXAMPLE of nonmaleficence?

A. Using expired meds
B. Skipping identity checks
C. Double-checking high-risk medications to prevent harm
D. Ignoring patient complaints

134.

A PATIENT SAYS, "MY pain is an 8/10 but you're not doing anything." The CMA's best response is:

A. "You're exaggerating."
B. "I'm sorry you're in pain. I'll let the provider know right away and see what we can do."
C. "Pain is normal."
D. "Deal with it."

135.

A PATIENT FREQUENTLY misses appointments. The CMA should:

A. Call them lazy
B. Dismiss them immediately
C. Use professional, non-judgmental language and follow policy for reminders and possible discharge
D. Charge random fees

136.

WHICH OF THE FOLLOWING is **NOT** appropriate to post on social media as a CMA?

A. A general article about handwashing
B. A vague complaint about "that diabetic in room 4" you had today
C. A link to the clinic's public flu clinic announcement
D. A reminder to get vaccines (no PHI)

137.

FOR A CAPILLARY FINGERSTICK, which finger(s) are typically used in adults?

A. Thumb
B. Index or middle finger (lateral side)
C. Pinky only
D. Palm

138.

EXCESSIVE SQUEEZING ("milking") of a finger during capillary collection can cause:

A. Hemolysis and inaccurate results
B. Better circulation
C. Less pain
D. Stronger nails

139.

ORDER OF DRAW AWARENESS helps:

A. Prevent cross-contamination of additives
B. Reduce patient anxiety
C. Improve office décor
D. Avoid billing errors

140.

THE **primary** purpose of a requisition form with a specimen is to:

A. Provide decoration
B. Identify what tests are ordered and link specimen to patient and provider
C. Replace labels
D. Track staff break times

141.

A RAPID FLU TEST IS negative, but the patient clearly appears severely ill with respiratory distress. The CMA should:

A. Assume they are fine
B. Rely only on the test result
C. Recognize that clinical status matters; notify provider of symptoms despite negative test
D. Send them home automatically

142.

PEAK FLOW READINGS are used primarily to monitor:

A. Heart function
B. Lung function in conditions like asthma
C. Kidney function
D. Brain function

143.

A PATIENT DECLINES a recommended vaccine after education. The CMA should:

A. Sneak the vaccine in anyway
B. Document the refusal and notify the provider
C. Yell at the patient
D. Discharge them immediately

144.

WHICH PEDIATRIC VITAL sign is normally higher than adults?

A. Blood pressure
B. Heart rate and respiratory rate
C. Height
D. Spine temperature

145.

A 6-YEAR-OLD IS NERVOUS about an injection. The CMA's best approach is:

A. "Don't be a baby."
B. Use simple explanations, offer comfort, and possibly distraction (like counting or toys)
C. Threaten punishment
D. Ignore their feelings

146.

WHICH SIGN MAY SUGGEST elder abuse or neglect?

A. Good hygiene
B. Multiple unexplained bruises and poor hygiene
C. Regular appointment attendance
D. Appropriate clothing

147.

WHEN SUSPECTED ABUSE is present, the CMA should:

A. Prove it personally
B. Document observations objectively and follow mandatory reporting policy
C. Confront the accused in public
D. Ignore it

148.

ORTHOSTATIC VITAL SIGNS are taken to evaluate:

A. Fever
B. Blood pressure changes with position, often related to dizziness/falls
C. Blood sugar
D. Allergies

149.

A PATIENT WITH COPD should be advised to:

A. Avoid all activity
B. Smoke occasionally
C. Follow provider's breathing treatment plan and use inhalers as instructed
D. Ignore symptoms

150.

WHICH IS A SIGN OF **respiratory distress**?

A. Speaking full sentences easily
B. Normal respiratory rate
C. Use of accessory muscles and inability to speak in full sentences
D. Quiet, regular breathing

151.

A PATIENT SCHEDULED for spirometry should be instructed to:

A. Eat a heavy meal immediately beforehand
B. Take a deep breath and blow forcefully into the device as instructed
C. Whisper into the device
D. Cough repeatedly into the device

152.

SUTURE REMOVAL MAY be performed by a CMA:

A. Only when self-prescribed
B. Under provider order and per policy/training
C. Never in any setting
D. Without gloves

153.

WHICH WOUND FINDING should be reported promptly?

A. Edges well approximated
B. Slight tenderness only
C. Wound edges gaping with active bleeding
D. Dry, intact dressing

154.

POSITIONING FOR A PELVIC exam is usually:

A. Sims'
B. Lithotomy
C. Fowler's
D. Prone

155.

BEFORE INTIMATE PROCEDURES, the CMA should:

A. Leave the door open
B. Provide gown/drape, explain procedure, and ensure privacy
C. Make jokes
D. Avoid explanation

156.

IN ADMINISTERING OXYGEN, the CMA's role is typically to:

A. Decide the liter flow without order
B. Apply oxygen as ordered and monitor patient's status, reporting concerns
C. Prescribe long-term oxygen
D. Change device type without provider input

157.

WHICH IS **most appropriate** when a patient speaks little English and no interpreter is available immediately for a non-emergent visit?

A. Use family children to interpret complex topics
B. Use interpreter services by phone/video per policy
C. Proceed with no communication
D. Make them sign a waiver

158.

A PATIENT'S CHART NOTES "allergic to latex." The CMA should:

A. Use latex gloves anyway
B. Use non-latex supplies and alert others as needed
C. Ignore it if no rash is seen
D. Ask the patient to bring their own gloves

159.

A PATIENT REFUSES TO allow a student CMA to participate in their care. The CMA should:

A. Force the student on them
B. Respect the refusal and assign tasks accordingly
C. Discharge the patient
D. Ignore the request

160.

A PATIENT INSISTS ON recording the visit with their phone. The CMA should:

A. Allow it without question
B. Throw the phone away
C. Follow clinic policy on recording in clinical areas and involve provider/manager as needed
D. Secretly record them back

161.

THE CMA IS CHARTING and realizes they are documenting in the wrong patient's EHR. They should:

A. Continue anyway

B. Delete all entries with no note

C. Correct the error following EHR policy (e.g., amend or mark as entered in error) and re-enter under correct patient

D. Ignore it

162.

A PATIENT SAYS THEY sometimes cut their pills in half to save money. The CMA should:

A. Approve it automatically

B. Explain that changing doses should only be done under provider direction and notify provider about cost concerns

C. Tell them to cut all pills

D. Ignore

163.

WHICH LAB TEST IS COMMONLY used to monitor long-term glucose control in diabetes?

A. CBC

B. Hemoglobin A1c

C. PT/INR

D. Lipid panel

164.

A CAPILLARY BLOOD GLUCOSE reading is extremely high, but the meter failed QC that morning. The CMA should:

A. Report the number as accurate

B. Recognize the meter is unreliable; repeat using a working device or send to lab per policy and notify provider

C. Guess a normal value

D. Ignore the result

165.

A PATIENT ON ANTICOAGULANT therapy reports black, tarry stools. The CMA should:

A. Consider it normal

B. Notify the provider immediately due to possible GI bleeding

C. Recommend more iron

D. Ignore

166.

WHICH IS A **red-flag symptom** of possible myocardial infarction?

A. Mild, brief twinge once

B. Crushing chest pain radiating to arm/jaw with diaphoresis

C. Itchy skin
D. Mild earache

167.

WHICH EKG ARTIFACT is most likely caused by patient shivering?
A. Somatic tremor
B. AC interference
C. Wandering baseline
D. Flat line

168.

AN EKG LEAD IS PLACED over thick chest hair and won't adhere well. The CMA should:
A. Tape it loosely
B. Remove or trim hair as allowed by policy and reapply electrode
C. Use glue
D. Place lead on clothing

169.

A PATIENT COMPLAINS of burning, frequent urination. The CMA should suspect involvement of which system?
A. Respiratory
B. Urinary
C. Musculoskeletal
D. Nervous

170.

BRIGHT RED BLOOD ON toilet tissue after a bowel movement might suggest:
A. Upper GI bleed
B. Hemorrhoids or lower rectal bleeding
C. Healthy digestion
D. Normal thirst

171.

PATIENT TEACHING FOR constipation prevention often includes:
A. Low fiber, reduced fluids
B. Adequate fluids, fiber, and activity as tolerated
C. Complete bed rest
D. Avoid fruits and vegetables

172.

A PATIENT PRESENTS with yellowing of skin and eyes (jaundice). This is often associated with which organ?
A. Heart
B. Liver

C. Kidney
D. Thyroid

173.

WHICH IS CONSIDERED PHI and must be protected?
A. Clinic lobby photo with no patients identifiable
B. Patient's name and diagnosis together
C. Generic health infographic
D. Weather report

174.

A PATIENT ASKS WHAT "NPO after midnight" means. The CMA should say:
A. "Only coffee and water after midnight."
B. "Nothing to eat or drink after midnight."
C. "Snack lightly."
D. "Skip only solids."

175.

A PATIENT SCHEDULED for a procedure is NPO but is observed drinking a large soda in the waiting room. The CMA should:
A. Ignore it
B. Inform provider or nurse, as the procedure may need to be delayed or rescheduled
C. Take the soda and drink it
D. Proceed as planned

176.

A PATIENT CALLS SAYING they took double their blood pressure medication by mistake and feels dizzy. The CMA should:
A. Say "you'll be fine"
B. Advise them per office triage protocol, which may include calling EMS or speaking to provider immediately
C. Tell them to sleep it off
D. Refuse advice

177.

WHICH IS AN EXAMPLE of **subjective** documentation?
A. BP 150/90 mmHg
B. "Patient reports nausea and 'stomach feels queasy.'"
C. Pulse 90 bpm
D. Wound 2 cm in length

178.

"WNL" IN CHARTING TYPICALLY means:

A. With no limit
B. Within normal limits
C. Will not last
D. With new labs

179.

A PATIENT IS EXTREMELY anxious about test results and calls repeatedly. The CMA should:
A. Ignore calls
B. Provide calm reassurance, explain process/timeline, and notify provider of frequent concerns
C. Yell at patient to stop calling
D. Give random guesses

180.

A COWORKER IS HEARD sharing patient details in the elevator. The CMA should:
A. Join in
B. Ignore
C. Remind them privately this is not appropriate and may violate confidentiality, and consider reporting if repeated
D. Record and post online

181.

A PATIENT SAYS THEY use someone else's prescription pain pills when theirs run out. The CMA should:
A. Approve
B. Explain the risks of sharing medications and notify providers of misuse concerns
C. Ignore
D. Ask for some

182.

A PATIENT WITH A NEW cast reports tingling, increased pain, and cold fingers distal to the cast. The CMA should:
A. Consider it normal
B. Notify provider immediately; possible circulation compromise
C. Recommend more rest only
D. Ignore

183.

THE CMA IS PREPARING to send a specimen to an outside lab. Which is essential?
A. No label needed
B. Properly labeled specimen, completed requisition, and correct packaging per lab instructions
C. Verbal note only
D. Sending it in a plain envelope

184.

A DISGRUNTLED PATIENT asks the CMA for the provider's personal phone number. The CMA should:

A. Give it
B. Politely decline and provide appropriate office contact methods
C. Make one up
D. Share their own

185.

A PATIENT CONTINUES to ask the same question repeatedly in one visit. The CMA should:

A. Show impatience
B. Repeat explanations calmly, check understanding, and ensure information is clear
C. Walk out
D. Mock them

186.

A CHILD WITH FEVER and a stiff neck is very lethargic. The CMA should:

A. Treat as routine
B. Notify provider immediately—possible serious infection
C. Send home
D. Offer candy

187.

A PATIENT SAYS, "I sometimes think everyone would be better off without me." The CMA should:

A. Ignore comment
B. Take it seriously, ensure the provider is notified immediately, and follow office protocol for mental health/suicide risk
C. Joke about it
D. Tell them not to mention it

188.

A PATIENT WITH A KNOWN latex allergy is scheduled for minor surgery. The CMA's role includes:

A. Using standard latex supplies
B. Ensuring latex-free supplies are available and flagging allergy to the team
C. Changing diagnosis
D. Ignoring allergy

189.

THE CMA NOTICES A STRONG smell of alcohol on a coworker's breath at 9 a.m. The coworker is about to start patient care. The CMA should:

A. Ignore it
B. Joke with them
C. Report concerns immediately per facility policy (impaired staff)
D. Take over their patients secretly

190.

A PATIENT REPORTS THEY take double their prescribed anxiety medication when stressed. The CMA should:

A. Approve
B. Explain medications should be taken only as prescribed and notify provider of this information
C. Suggest tripling dose
D. Ignore

191.

A PATIENT COMPLAINS that the CMA is "rude and uncaring." The most professional response is to:

A. Argue with the patient
B. Listen calmly, apologize for any misunderstanding, and refer concern to supervisor if needed
C. Mock the patient
D. Walk away

192.

WHICH IS AN EXAMPLE of **professional appearance** for a CMA?

A. Strong perfume, wrinkled clothes
B. Clean uniform, minimal jewelry, name badge, and good hygiene
C. Pajamas
D. Dirty shoes

193.

A PATIENT WANTS TO pay cash and asks not to bill insurance for a covered service. The CMA should:

A. Automatically agree
B. Follow office policy and possibly consult billing/management regarding legal/contractual obligations
C. Hide it
D. Refuse care

194.

A PATIENT'S BLOOD SPECIMEN hemolyzes due to vigorous shaking. The CMA should:

A. Report the inaccurate result as is
B. Recognize it may be invalid and recollect if ordered, using proper technique
C. Guess values
D. Ignore

195.

A PATIENT IS NPO AND asks if they can chew gum. The CMA should:

A. Say "yes, gum is fine"
B. Explain that chewing gum may stimulate gastric secretions and typically is not allowed; verify per provider/policy
C. Tell them to chew a lot
D. Ignore

196.

WHEN USING AN AUTOCLAVE, the **most important** factor to ensure proper sterilization is:

A. Color of the machine

B. Correct time, temperature, and pressure according to guidelines

C. How loud it is

D. Size of the room

197.

STERILIZATION DIFFERS from disinfection because sterilization:

A. Only cleans visible dirt

B. Kills all forms of microbial life, including spores

C. Is less effective than disinfection

D. Only uses cold water

198.

A PATIENT WITH A NEW diagnosis asks, “Will searching online tell me everything I need?” The CMA should:

A. Say yes, internet is all you need

B. Suggest reliable sources and emphasize discussing findings with the provider

C. Forbid internet use

D. Provide random blogs

199.

A PATIENT BECOMES VERY quiet and withdrawn when a certain family member enters the room. The CMA’s best action is to:

A. Ignore it

B. Document observations and, if concerned, notify provider about possible safety or abuse concerns

C. Confront the family member publicly

D. Ask no one

200.

A PATIENT ASKS THE CMA to change information in the chart to hide a prior diagnosis from an insurer. The CMA should:

A. Agree to alter the record

B. Refuse and explain records must be accurate and complete, and refer them to provider/office manager for questions

C. Delete diagnoses secretly

D. Take cash for changes

Answer Key with Justifications and Section References

1. **C** – Fasting status is compromised; provider/lab must decide. *(Ch 7.3 Specimen Collection: Urine & Blood)*
2. **C** – Administering ordered meds is in scope; prescribing/altering doses is not. *(Ch 6.1 CMA's Role in Medication Management)*
3. **B** – Allergy + related drug requires clarification before giving. *(Ch 6.7 High-Alert Meds & Allergies)*
4. **B** – Subjective = patient-reported feelings. *(Ch 4.4 Documentation & Data Types)*
5. **B** – Two identifiers compared to orders is standard. *(Ch 7.2 Patient Identification & Safety)*
6. **B** – Label in patient's presence immediately after collection. *(Ch 7.3 Specimen Collection)*
7. **A** – First sound = systolic; disappearance = diastolic. *(Ch 3.3 Vital Signs – Blood Pressure)*
8. **B** – Turning away breaks sterility. *(Ch 8.2 Sterile Fields & Aseptic Technique)*
9. **B** – Stop drawing, protect the patient from fainting-related injury. *(Ch 7.4 Blood Collection Safety)*
10. **C** – Unlabeled specimens must be discarded and recollected. *(Ch 7.3 Specimen Collection)*
11. **C** – Chest pain + SOB is an emergency red flag. *(Ch 13.4 Clinical Reasoning & Priorities)*
12. **C** – Clean, start in the toilet, then collect midstream. *(Ch 7.3 Specimen Collection: Urine)*
13. **B** – Verify identity and follow policy/provider direction. *(Ch 5.3 Phone Etiquette & Results)*
14. **B** – PHI is any identifiable health info in any form. *(Ch 12.3 Confidentiality & HIPAA)*
15. **B** – True informed consent requires explanation + voluntary agreement. *(Ch 12.2 Informed Consent)*
16. **B** – Unsafe abbreviation must be clarified and rewritten. *(Ch 6.4 Med Orders & Rights; Ch 11.8 High-Risk Abbrev.)*
17. **B** – All substances matter for interactions. *(Ch 6.7 High-Alert Medications & Allergies; Ch 9.7 Polypharmacy)*
18. **B** – Wheezing/exhalation difficulty = respiratory system. *(Ch 10.5 Respiratory System)*
19. **C** – "Poly-" = many/excessive; "-uria" = urine. *(Ch 11.6 Number & Size Prefixes)*
20. **B** – High fever + lethargy + poor intake in a toddler is urgent. *(Ch 9.3 Pediatric Vitals & Safety)*
21. **B** – Fix electrode issue and repeat EKG. *(Ch 7.6 ECG Basics)*
22. **B** – CMA can calculate/record BMI; provider interprets. *(Ch 3.4 Anthropometrics & BMI)*
23. **C** – PO = by mouth. *(Ch 11.7 Common Abbreviations)*
24. **B** – New confusion is concerning and must be reported. *(Ch 9.6 Geriatric Assessment)*
25. **C** – Objective, quotes patient, notes provider notification. *(Ch 4.4 Documentation & Objectivity)*
26. **B** – Pale, shaky, sweaty = likely hypoglycemia. *(Ch 6.6 Medication Safety & Awareness)*
27. **B** – Abdomen SC site is appropriate per policy. *(Ch 6.5 Routes of Administration)*
28. **A** – Gloves are standard for blood exposure. *(Ch 4.3 PPE & Standard Precautions)*
29. **B** – Respect confidentiality per law/policy. *(Ch 12.3 Confidentiality & PHI)*
30. **B** – Unsafe failure to secure child = negligence. *(Ch 12.5 Negligence & Liability)*
31. **B** – Possible developmental delay; document and notify provider. *(Ch 9.2 Pediatric Development & Communication)*
32. **B** – Acknowledge feelings, explain, protect privacy. *(Ch 9.9 Obstetric/Gyn Sensitivity; Ch 7.9 Intimate Procedures)*
33. **B** – Do not perform untrained tasks; request training. *(Ch 12.1 Scope of Practice & Delegation)*
34. **D** – QID = four times daily. *(Ch 11.7 Timing Abbreviations)*
35. **B** – Classic pregnancy warning signs; urgent. *(Ch 9.8 Obstetric Assessment)*
36. **C** – Always clarify unclear orders. *(Ch 6.4 Orders & Rights; Ch 12.10 Reporting Safety Issues)*
37. **C** – Interpretation is the provider's role; CMA facilitates. *(Ch 11.10 Patient-Friendly Language & Scope)*

38. **B** – Immediate washing and exposure protocol. *(Ch 4.3 Standard Precautions & OSHA)*
39. **B** – Standard precautions apply to all patients based on exposure risk. *(Ch 4.2 Infection Control Principles)*
40. **A** – Basic life support chain: check, call, activate response. *(Ch 8.7 BLS & AED)*
41. **B** – Suggests fall risk; document and notify provider. *(Ch 9.7 Geriatric Safety & Functional Status)*
42. **B** – "Hepat-" = liver; "-itis" = inflammation. *(Ch 11.2 System Roots)*
43. **B** – "Brady-" = slow; "cardia" = heart. *(Ch 11.6 Number/Speed Prefixes)*
44. **C** – Complete, objective description of procedure. *(Ch 4.4 Documentation)*
45. **C** – Possible stroke; treat as emergency. *(Ch 13.4 Clinical Reasoning – Red Flags)*
46. **B** – Significant BP change must be reported. *(Ch 3.3 Vital Signs – BP)*
47. **B** – Replace expired meds and report the lapse. *(Ch 8.9 Emergency Equipment Readiness)*
48. **B** – "-ectomy" = removal; cholecystectomy = gallbladder removal. *(Ch 11.5 Procedure Suffixes)*
49. **B** – Stay calm, acknowledge, and help. *(Ch 5.2 Professional Communication with Patients)*
50. **B** – Suspected abuse requires objective documentation and reporting. *(Ch 9.5 Child Abuse & Reporting; Ch 12.10 Reporting)*
51. **C** – Provider must ensure understanding; CMA alerts them. *(Ch 12.2 Informed Consent)*
52. **C** – "Daily" avoids confusion; QD/OD are risky. *(Ch 11.8 High-Risk Abbreviations)*
53. **B** – Critical values require read-back and urgent provider notification. *(Ch 7.10 Result Reporting & Follow-Up)*
54. **B** – Clear, accurate vaccine explanation. *(Ch 6.8 & 6.10 Immunizations & Teaching)*
55. **B** – Encourages correct schedule and safe response to missed doses. *(Ch 6.10 Patient Education – Meds)*
56. **C** – Impaired staff endanger patients; follow policy. *(Ch 12.10 Reporting Unsafe Conditions)*
57. **B** – Sympathetic system = fight or flight. *(Ch 10.6 Nervous System)*
58. **B** – Ask preferences; avoid stereotypes. *(Ch 12.7 Cultural Competence)*
59. **B** – Teaching and return demonstration are in scope. *(Ch 7.7 Pulmonary Testing & Resp. Teaching)*
60. **B** – Acknowledge feelings, clarify key points, ensure access. *(Ch 13.7 Ethics & Communication)*
61. **B** – Standard precautions for all based on exposure. *(Ch 4.2 Infection Control)*
62. **B** – Droplet = surgical mask near coughing patient. *(Ch 4.2 Transmission-Based Precautions)*
63. **B** – Hand hygiene reduces microorganism spread. *(Ch 4.3 Hand Hygiene)*
64. **C** – Mosquito is a vector. *(Ch 4.1 Infection Chain)*
65. **C** – Common recommendation: ~15–20 seconds friction. *(Ch 4.3 Hand Hygiene)*
66. **C** – Sharps go in sharps containers only. *(Ch 4.3 Sharps Safety)*
67. **B** – QC ensures reliable patient results. *(Ch 7.5 POCT & QC)*
68. **B** – Reading outside the time window risks false results. *(Ch 7.5 POCT Timing)*
69. **C** – Infectious agent is the first link. *(Ch 4.1 Chain of Infection)*
70. **C** – Big jump in RR with dyspnea suggests distress. *(Ch 3.2 Respirations)*
71. **B** – Normal adult RR ~12–20/min. *(Ch 3.2 Respirations)*
72. **B** – Radial pulse commonly used in adults. *(Ch 3.1 Pulse)*
73. **C** – BMI uses height and weight. *(Ch 3.4 BMI)*
74. **B** – Severe asthma distress is an emergency. *(Ch 10.5 Respiratory; Ch 13.4 Priorities)*
75. **A** – CNS: brain + spinal cord. *(Ch 10.6 Nervous System)*
76. **B** – Thyroid = metabolism. *(Ch 10.7 Endocrine)*
77. **B** – The small intestine is the main absorption site. *(Ch 10.8 Digestive System)*
78. **B** – Kidneys filter blood and form urine. *(Ch 10.9 Urinary System)*
79. **B** – Erythema = redness. *(Ch 10.10 Integumentary)*

80. **A** – Ligaments connect bone to bone. *(Ch 10.10 Musculoskeletal)*
81. **B** – Classic local infection signs. *(Ch 8.8 Wound Care & Infection)*
82. **B** – Side-lying/Sims' is common for rectal temp. *(Ch 3.1 Temperature & Positioning)*
83. **A** – Adult deltoid injections commonly use ~1–1.5" needles. *(Ch 6.5 Routes & Technique)*
84. **C** – Temperature excursion compromises vaccine; discard per policy. *(Ch 6.9 Vaccine Storage)*
85. **B** – Mild soreness/low fever are expected minor reactions. *(Ch 6.10 Vaccine Teaching)*
86. **B** – Proper vaccine documentation list. *(Ch 6.8–6.9 Immunization Documentation)*
87. **B** – Refusal must be documented and shared with the provider. *(Ch 12.2 Consent & Refusal)*
88. **A** – Advance directives guide care if a patient can't decide. *(Ch 12.9 Patient Rights & Advance Directives)*
89. **B** – DNR = Do Not Resuscitate. *(Ch 12.9)*
90. **C** – Private, respectful conflict resolution focused on care. *(Ch 12.8 Professionalism & Teamwork)*
91. **C** – Friendly but care-focused maintains boundaries. *(Ch 12.7 Professional Boundaries)*
92. **B** – Incident reports support safety/improvement. *(Ch 12.10 Incident Reporting)*
93. **B** – c/o = complains of. *(Ch 11.9 Chart Shorthand)*
94. **A** – SOB = shortness of breath. *(Ch 11.7 & 11.9)*
95. **B** – Hyperglycemia = high blood sugar. *(Ch 10.7 Endocrine/Diabetes)*
96. **A** – Gastritis = stomach inflammation. *(Ch 11.4 Pathology Suffixes)*
97. **B** – "-ectomy" = removal; nephrectomy = kidney removal. *(Ch 11.5)*
98. **A** – Benign = non-cancerous growth. *(Ch 11.10 Patient-Friendly Explanations)*
99. **C** – "U" is easily misread; unsafe. *(Ch 11.8 High-Risk Abbrev.)*
100. **C** – Single line, mark error, initial/date, correct. *(Ch 4.4 Documentation Correction Rules)*
101. **C** – Direct to appropriate billing resource; don't guess. *(Ch 5.4 Financial Comms)*
102. **B** – Triage prioritizes by severity/urgency. *(Ch 5.1 Front Desk & Triage)*
103. **B** – Professional phone greeting with identification. *(Ch 5.3 Phone Etiquette)*
104. **B** – Demographic info should be updated accurately. *(Ch 5.1 Registration & EHR)*
105. **A** – Wave scheduling: same-time arrivals seen in order. *(Ch 5.2 Scheduling Systems)*
106. **B** – Stream = evenly spaced appointments. *(Ch 5.2)*
107. **B** – Tickler = reminder/follow-up system. *(Ch 5.5 Record & Reminder Systems)*
108. **B** – Provide payment options; follow policy and document. *(Ch 5.4 Collections & Payments)*
109. **B** – Correct/complete claim data and resubmit. *(Ch 5.6 Billing & Claims)*
110. **B** – Verify fax number, use cover sheet, follow policy. *(Ch 12.3 HIPAA & PHI Transmission)*
111. **B** – Limit public info to what policy allows (name/time). *(Ch 12.3 & 5.1)*
112. **C** – Subpoenas handled per legal/records policy. *(Ch 12.4 Medical Records & Law)*
113. **C** – Follow disruptive behavior policy; ensure safety. *(Ch 12.8 Professionalism & Safety)*
114. **B** – Neutral, professional phrasing for copay. *(Ch 5.4)*
115. **C** – Follow formal release process. *(Ch 12.4 Records Access)*
116. **B** – Explain in plain language; provider for clinical details. *(Ch 11.10 & 5.1)*
117. **B** – Financial corrections similar to clinical: single line + initials/date. *(Ch 5.6 Basic Bookkeeping)*
118. **C** – Follow office late-arrival policy. *(Ch 5.2 Scheduling)*
119. **B** – ICD codes classify diagnoses. *(Ch 5.7 Coding Basics)*
120. **B** – CPT codes describe procedures/services. *(Ch 5.7)*
121. **B** – Modifier adds detail to procedure code. *(Ch 5.7)*
122. **B** – Hemoptysis after surgery may indicate serious bleeding. *(Ch 7.10 Reporting Results & Symptoms)*
123. **B** – Insulin changes need a provider; notify about concern. *(Ch 6.10 Med Teaching & Safety)*

124. **B** – Use qualified interpreter services when possible. *(Ch 12.7 Cultural Competence & Communication)*
125. **B** – Teach-back = patient repeats in own words. *(Ch 11.10 & 13.7)*
126. **B** – Document refusal and follow ABN/insurer policy. *(Ch 5.6 Insurance & ABNs)*
127. **B** – OSHA protects workers from hazards. *(Ch 4.3 OSHA & Exposure Control)*
128. **B** – Safety needles are engineering controls. *(Ch 4.3 Exposure Controls)*
129. **B** – Exposure plan must be written and accessible. *(Ch 4.3 OSHA Requirements)*
130. **D** – Autonomy = respect for patient decisions. *(Ch 12.6 Ethics – Autonomy)*
131. **A** – Beneficence = doing good for patient welfare. *(Ch 12.6 Ethics)*
132. **B** – Justice = fairness/equity in care. *(Ch 12.6 Ethics)*
133. **C** – Double-checking meds prevents harm (nonmaleficence). *(Ch 12.6 & 6.6)*
134. **B** – Acknowledge pain and act by informing the provider. *(Ch 13.7 Communication & Ethics)*
135. **C** – Use professional language and follow office policies. *(Ch 12.8 Professionalism)*
136. **B** – Even without name, referencing "diabetic in room 4" risks PHI; unprofessional. *(Ch 12.3 & 12.7 Social Media)*
137. **B** – Lateral side of index/middle finger for adults. *(Ch 7.4 Capillary Testing)*
138. **A** – Excessive squeezing can hemolyze samples. *(Ch 7.4 Blood Collection)*
139. **A** – Order of draw prevents additive cross-contamination. *(Ch 7.4 Lab Safety)*
140. **B** – Requisition links specimen, tests, and provider. *(Ch 7.3–7.4)*
141. **C** – Clinical picture overrides single negative POCT; notify provider. *(Ch 7.5 POCT & Clinical Correlation)*
142. **B** – Peak flow monitors lung function. *(Ch 7.7 Pulmonary Testing)*
143. **B** – Document refusal and inform the provider. *(Ch 6.10 & 12.2)*
144. **B** – Pediatric HR and RR are typically higher than adults. *(Ch 9.3 Pediatric Vitals)*
145. **B** – Age-appropriate explanation and comfort/distraction. *(Ch 9.1–9.2 Pediatric Care)*
146. **B** – Multiple unexplained bruises + poor hygiene can suggest abuse/neglect. *(Ch 9.5 Geriatric/Elder Abuse)*
147. **B** – Suspected abuse = objective documentation + mandatory reporting. *(Ch 9.5 & 12.10)*
148. **B** – Orthostatics evaluate BP changes with position. *(Ch 3.3 Vital Signs – Orthostatic)*
149. **C** – Follow ordered breathing treatments and inhaler use. *(Ch 7.7 & 10.5)*
150. **C** – Accessory muscle use + limited speech = distress. *(Ch 10.5 & 13.4)*
151. **B** – Deep breath, forceful exhalation per spirometry instructions. *(Ch 7.7)*
152. **B** – Suture removal can be delegated per order/policy. *(Ch 8.8 Minor Office Procedures)*
153. **C** – Gaping with active bleeding is concerning. *(Ch 8.8 Wound Assessment)*
154. **B** – Lithotomy position for pelvic exams. *(Ch 7.9 & 9.9)*
155. **B** – Provide gown/drape, explanation, and privacy. *(Ch 7.9 Intimate Procedures)*
156. **B** – CMA applies oxygen as ordered and monitors; does not independently order. *(Ch 8.6 & 8.7 Emergencies)*
157. **B** – Use proper interpreter services. *(Ch 12.7 Cultural Competence)*
158. **B** – Use latex-free supplies and flag allergy. *(Ch 6.7 Allergies & Safety)*
159. **B** – Respect the patient's right to refuse student involvement. *(Ch 12.9 Patient Rights)*
160. **C** – Follow clinic policy about recording. *(Ch 12.3 Privacy & Clinic Policies)*
161. **C** – Correct EHR errors per policy and chart under correct patient. *(Ch 4.4 EHR Documentation)*
162. **B** – Dose changes require a provider; notify about cost issues. *(Ch 6.10 Med Education)*
163. **B** – HbA1c monitors long-term glucose control. *(Ch 10.7 Endocrine/Diabetes Basics)*
164. **B** – Failed QC = unreliable device; repeat using valid method. *(Ch 7.5 POCT QC)*
165. **B** – Black, tarry stools with anticoagulants suggest GI bleed; urgent. *(Ch 10.8 Digestive; Ch 13.4 Priorities)*
166. **B** – Classic MI symptom cluster. *(Ch 10.4 Cardiovascular; Ch 13.4)*

167. **A** – Somatic tremor artifact comes from muscle movement/shivering. *(Ch 7.6 ECG Artifacts)*
168. **B** – Remove/trim hair as allowed, reapply electrodes. *(Ch 7.6 ECG Prep)*
169. **B** – Dysuria/frequency involves the urinary system. *(Ch 10.9 Urinary)*
170. **B** – Bright red blood with wiping suggests hemorrhoids/lower rectal source. *(Ch 10.8 Digestive)*
171. **B** – Fluids, fiber, and movement help prevent constipation. *(Ch 10.8 + Patient Teaching)*
172. **B** – Jaundice strongly linked to liver/biliary disease. *(Ch 10.8)*
173. **B** – Name + diagnosis is PHI. *(Ch 12.3 PHI)*
174. **B** – NPO = nothing by mouth. *(Ch 11.7 & 6.4 Orders)*
175. **B** – NPO violation may require delaying/rescheduling; notify provider. *(Ch 13.4 Integrated Safety)*
176. **B** – Double dosing with dizziness needs triage/protocol and possible urgent care. *(Ch 6.6 Med Safety & 13.4)*
177. **B** – Subjective = patient's description. *(Ch 4.4 Subjective vs Objective)*
178. **B** – WNL = within normal limits. *(Ch 11.9 Shorthand)*
179. **B** – Calm explanation, clear timeline, and provider notification. *(Ch 5.3 & 13.7 Communication)*
180. **C** – Quiet reminder + possible reporting if ongoing. *(Ch 12.3 Confidentiality & Professionalism)*
181. **B** – Medication sharing is unsafe; providers must be informed. *(Ch 6.6–6.7 Med Safety)*
182. **B** – Signs of neurovascular compromise under cast. *(Ch 10.10 Musculoskeletal & 13.4)*
183. **B** – Label, requisition, proper packaging are essential. *(Ch 7.3–7.4 Specimen Handling)*
184. **B** – Protect boundaries; use official contact channels. *(Ch 12.7 Professional Boundaries)*
185. **B** – The patient may be anxious or confused; repeat calmly and check understanding. *(Ch 13.7 Communication)*
186. **B** – Fever + stiff neck + lethargy = possible meningitis; urgent. *(Ch 13.4 Red Flags)*
187. **B** – Suicidal statements must be taken seriously; follow mental health protocol. *(Ch 12.10 Reporting / Special Situations)*
188. **B** – Latex allergy requires latex-free setup and communication. *(Ch 6.7)*
189. **C** – Impaired staff must be reported per policy. *(Ch 12.10 Reporting Unsafe Conditions)*
190. **B** – Med misuse must be addressed and provider informed. *(Ch 6.6 Med Safety)*
191. **B** – Listen, apologize for experience, and escalate concern if needed. *(Ch 12.8 Professional Behavior)*
192. **B** – Clean uniform, minimal jewelry, good hygiene reflect professionalism. *(Ch 2.x Professional Image – from your earlier structure/Admin domain)*
193. **B** – Follow policy; there may be insurer contract rules. *(Ch 5.6 Billing & Ethics)*
194. **B** – Hemolyzed specimens are often invalid; recollect if needed. *(Ch 7.4 Specimen Quality)*
195. **B** – Gum may violate NPO rules; check policy/provider. *(Ch 13.4 Practical Safety Applications)*
196. **B** – Sterilization requires correct time/temperature/pressure. *(Ch 4.5 Sterilization & Disinfection)*
197. **B** – Sterilization kills all forms including spores; disinfection does not. *(Ch 4.5)*
198. **B** – Direct to reliable sources and provider discussion. *(Ch 11.10 & 13.7 Patient Education)*
199. **B** – Subtle behavior changes may indicate safety issues; observe, document, and notify the provider. *(Ch 9.5 Abuse & 13.4)*
200. **B** – Records must be accurate; refer to provider/manager for concerns, never falsify. *(Ch 12.4 Legal Records & Ethics)*

About the Author

CertiPrep Publishing specializes in high-quality certification exam prep books. We empower learners with expert resources to succeed in their professional certifications.

www.ingramcontent.com/pod-product-compliance
Lightning Source LLC
LaVergne TN
LVHW082339200926
848481LV00012B/3396